An Evidence-Based Critique of Contemporary Psychoanalysis

An Evidence-Based Critique of Contemporary Psychoanalysis assesses the state of psychoanalysis in the 21st century. Joel Paris examines areas where analysis needs to develop a stronger scientific and clinical base, and to integrate its ideas with modern clinical psychology and psychiatry.

While psychoanalysis has declined as an independent discipline, it continues to play a major role in clinical thought. Paris explores the extent to which analysis has gained support from recent empirical research. He argues that it could revive its influence by establishing a stronger relationship to science, whilst looking at the state of current research. For clinical applications, he suggests while convincing evidence is lacking to support long-term treatment, brief psychoanalytic therapy, lasting for a few months, has been shown to be relatively effective for common mental disorders. For theory, Paris reviews changes in the psychoanalytic paradigm, most particularly the shift from a theory based largely on intrapsychic mechanisms to the more interpersonal approach of attachment theory. He also reviews the interfaces between psychoanalysis and other disciplines, ranging from "neuropsychoanalysis" to the incorporation of analytic theory into post-modern models popular in the humanities.

An Evidence-Based Critique of Contemporary Psychoanalysis concludes by examining the legacy of psychoanalysis and making recommendations for integration into broader psychological theory and psychotherapy. It will be of great interest to psychoanalysts, psychoanalytic psychotherapists, and scholars and practitioners across the mental health professions interested in the future and influence of the field.

Joel Paris is Emeritus Professor of Psychiatry and a former Department Chair at McGill University, Montreal, Canada. His research interest is in borderline personality disorder and he is author of over 200 peer-reviewed articles, more than 20 books, and over 50 book chapters.

Psychological Issues
Series Editor DAVID L. WOLITZKY

The basic mission of *Psychological Issues* is to contribute to the further development of psychoanalysis as a science, as a respected scholarly enterprise, as a theory of human behavior, and as a therapeutic method.

Over the past 50 years, the series has focused on fundamental aspects and foundations of psychoanalytic theory and clinical practice, as well as on work in related disciplines relevant to psychoanalysis. *Psychological Issues* does not aim to represent or promote a particular point of view. The contributions cover broad and integrative topics of vital interest to all psychoanalysts as well as to colleagues in related disciplines. They cut across particular schools of thought and tackle key issues, such as the philosophical underpinnings of psychoanalysis, psychoanalytic theories of motivation, conceptions of therapeutic action, the nature of unconscious mental functioning, psychoanalysis and social issues, and reports of original empirical research relevant to psychoanalysis. The authors often take a critical stance toward theories and offer a careful theoretical analysis and conceptual clarification of the complexities of theories and their clinical implications, drawing upon relevant empirical findings from psychoanalytic research as well as from research in related fields.

Series Editor David L. Wolitzky and the Editorial Board continues to invite contributions from social/behavioral sciences such as anthropology and sociology, from biological sciences such as physiology and the various brain sciences, and from scholarly humanistic disciplines such as philosophy, law, and ethics. Volumes 1–64 in this series were published by International Universities Press. Volumes 65–69 were published by Jason Aronson. For a full list of the titles published by Routledge in this series, please visit the Routledge website: www.routledge.com/Psychological-Issues/book-series/PSYCHISSUES

An Evidence-Based Critique of Contemporary Psychoanalysis

Research, Theory, and Clinical Practice

Joel Paris

Routledge
Taylor & Francis Group
LONDON AND NEW YORK

First published 2019
by Routledge
2 Park Square, Milton Park, Abingdon, Oxon OX14 4RN

and by Routledge
52 Vanderbilt Avenue, New York, NY 10017

Routledge is an imprint of the Taylor & Francis Group, an informa business

British Library Cataloguing-in-Publication Data
A catalogue record for this book is available from the British Library

Library of Congress Cataloging-in-Publication Data
Names: Paris, Joel, 1940– author.
Title: An evidence-based critique of contemporary psychoanalysis : research, theory, and clinical practice / Joel Paris.
Description: New York : Routledge, 2019. | Series: Psychological issues ; 81 | Includes bibliographical references and index.
Identifiers: LCCN 2018042341 (print) | LCCN 2018053721 (ebook) | ISBN 9780429020674 (Master) | ISBN 9780429668043 (Adobe) | ISBN 9780429665325 (ePub) | ISBN 9780429662607 (MobiPocket) | ISBN 9780367074258 (hardback : alk. paper) | ISBN 9780367074289 (pbk. : alk. paper) | ISBN 9780429020674 (ebk)
Subjects: LCSH: Psychoanalysis. | Psychotherapy. | Psychoanalysts.
Classification: LCC RC504 (ebook) | LCC RC504 .P38 2019 (print) | DDC 616.89/17—dc23
LC record available at https://lccn.loc.gov/2018042341

ISBN: 978-0-367-07425-8 (hbk)
ISBN: 978-0-367-07428-9 (pbk)
ISBN: 978-0-429-02067-4 (ebk)

Typeset in Times New Roman
by Apex CoVantage, LLC

This book is dedicated to the psychoanalysts who taught me how to listen to patients, and to the analysts who have moved into the scientific mainstream.

Contents

Acknowledgements

I owe a great debt to David L. Wolitzky, who read the entire manuscript, and who, in spite of disagreeing with some of my ideas, challenged me to strengthen the argument. Ron Feldman read most of the chapters and made many useful comments and suggestions. For an earlier draft of the book, I benefited from the input of Ned Shorter and Todd Dufresne.

Introduction

Why I have written this book

Psychoanalysis is a psychological theory and a method of therapy for mental disorders. It has had an enormous influence on modern culture. However its impact on academic and clinical disciplines has greatly declined.

I trained at a time when its ideas dominated much of psychiatry and clinical psychology. As a psychiatric resident in the late 1960s, many of my teachers were either trained psychoanalysts or psychodynamically oriented therapists. Yet while some of my mentors advised me to train in psychoanalysis, I did not apply to an analytic institute. I aimed to treat the sickest patients, and was interested in briefer therapies. Moreover, I was skeptical about the orthodoxy that plagued the field. Even so, the first half of my career was largely devoted to practicing psychodynamic psychotherapy, and teaching it to the next generation of residents. Colleagues from other institutions saw me that way, and assumed I was "one of them".

In many ways this trajectory was typical of my generation. I studied psychiatry when psychoanalysis was at its peak of its influence. At the time up to 10% of medical graduates chose psychiatry as a specialty (Tamaskar and McGinnis, 2002). Many of those who made this choice were inspired by the ideas of Freud and his followers.

Psychoanalysis was lengthy and expensive, but was often considered to be the "Rolls Royce" of psychotherapies. One reason was that, in spite of the proliferation of talking therapies, the competition was weak. Behavior therapy was narrow in theory and mechanistic in practice. Cognitive behavioral therapy (CBT) had not yet appeared on the scene.

But was psychoanalysis evidence-based? Like most psychiatrists, I had minimal training in research, and had to teach myself the principles of evidence-based practice. And for a long time I could not even see the relevance of research to psychological forms of treatment. As one of my colleagues quipped, "the most important questions are not researchable, and the most researchable questions are not important". Immersed in a culture that idealized psychoanalysis, I could not see how its insights into the psyche could be evaluated in empirical studies. I largely accepted the clinical methods by which psychoanalysts sought truth, reaching broad conclusions based on the intensive study of a small number of patients.

It took me 15 years to change my mind. By the 1980s, the role of psychoanalysis in academic psychiatry was in decline. A training analyst who led my hospital department for 25 years retired, and his successors were not committed to the cause. At the university level, analysts who had served as academic chairs of the department were replaced by researchers. I have described these trends in a previous book (Paris, 2005).

At the same time, CBT began to take over as the leading form of psychological treatment. Clinical psychologists, who usually had more training in the method, became the primary providers of psychotherapy. At the same time, psychiatry was moving away from all forms of psychotherapy, focusing on pharmacotherapy, sometimes defining itself as an "application of clinical neuroscience" (Insel and Quirion, 2005). Little by little, psychiatrists began to be seen, not as wizards of the psyche, but as having tools to correct "chemical imbalances" in the brain.

None of these changes would have shaken my views if I had been convinced that the years I spent applying a psychodynamic model to patients had been consistently fruitful. Like other therapists, I had successes and liked to talk about them. Yet some of my best results came from seeing patients for just a few months. I could not deny that some of those who I followed for years achieved little change.

This reflection on clinical experiences led me to reconsider my earlier lack of commitment to research. As an undergraduate, I had majored in psychology, but had not been taught investigative skills. Now I became interested in the idea that practice should be based, not on impressions drawn from clinical experience, or on theoretical considerations, but on empirical evidence showing that treatments actually work. Gradually, I became a "born again" convert to evidence-based practice. And although I had a late start (in my forties), I developed a second career as a researcher.

Working with PhD colleagues, I retrained myself to carry out empirical work. My clinical interests determined my focus, and I was able to get in on the ground floor of research on borderline personality disorder (BPD). This condition was of particular interest to psychoanalysts, but had long defied attempts to apply treatment effectively.

Becoming a clinical researcher, I developed a strong attachment to the cause of evidence-based practice, both in medicine (Sackett et al., 1996), and clinical psychology (APA Presidential Task Force on Evidence-Based Practice, 2006). By "evidence based", I mean treatment interventions supported by controlled trials and meta-analyses of research findings. This does not mean that I fail to recognize the limitations of research methods that have difficulty in measuring subjectivity. However I reject the idea that clinical experience, supported by case studies, is as good as or superior a method as empirical research. A good example of this view was an article in the *Journal of the American Psychoanalytic Association* (Hoffman, 2009). In a response published in the same journal, Eagle and Wolitsky (2011) pointed out that clinical experience, often shaped by preconceptions, all too often leads to incorrect conclusions, and that case histories, however powerful their narrative, tend to be afflicted by theoretical biases of all kinds.

Thus, even though I have practiced for five decades, I no longer trust my own experience. Instead, a shift to research led me to question many aspects of my work. Research leads to the conclusion that all psychotherapies should have a clear structure, focus on a goal, and be time-limited (Lambert, 2013). It also leads to the conclusion that most forms of effective psychotherapy work in the same way (Wampold, 2001). While I continue to use many psychodynamic principles, I have come to support an integrative psychotherapy that does not adhere to any school of thought. While research has not shown that an integrative approach necessarily achieves superior results, it seems commonsensical to make use of the best ideas from all sources.

What this book is about

This book presents a sympathetic but critical critique of contemporary psychoanalysis based on scientific principles. While clinical work cannot be guided in detail by the principle of evidence-based practice, it should at least be consistent with what research shows.

Psychoanalysis offered a great deal to mental health treatment, but has fallen behind the times. This book will not focus on the ideas of Sigmund

Freud, which are now a century old, and which have already undergone detailed criticism (e.g., MacMillan, 1991). Today these ideas have largely been supplanted by more modern approaches. Even so, both the theory of psychoanalysis and its clinical application need serious revision.

To this end, I will examine the place of psychoanalysis in 21st-century theory and practice. As the world changed, so did psychoanalysis. Its central ideas have gradually become less intrapsychic and more interpersonal and relational. Analytic therapy has evolved into a method to modify serious problems in managing and maintaining close relationships.

I will address the question as to whether formal psychoanalysis, several times a week for years, is the best way to provide psychological treatment. First, there is little convincing evidence that long-term therapy is necessary for most people clinicians see. Moreover, the theory and practice of psychodynamic therapy face serious competition from other approaches, such as CBT. Psychoanalysis could benefit from adapting its methods to make them more practical, and to integrate a psychodynamic approach into a broader model of psychotherapy.

Second, the expense of psychoanalysis makes it unavailable to most patients. This problem could be addressed by offering time-limited therapy with a lower frequency of sessions. Recent research shows that brief psychoanalytic therapy has strong efficacy, and that once weekly treatment, lasting for only a few months, can be effective in the treatment of many mental disorders (Leichsenring et al., 2004; Abbass et al., 2014). It is not widely known that most of Freud's patients were only seen for a few months. The later tradition of extended psychoanalysis over many years only grew up because a good number of patients did not improve in short-term treatment (Hale, 1995).

This book will show that research has not found good evidence to support the idea that extensive courses of therapy based on psychoanalysis produce results that cannot be obtained using briefer interventions. It follows that short-term treatment could be a default condition, and that long-term intervention could be reserved for cases where it proves insufficient. That would be an example of "stepped care" (Bower and Gilboody, 2005).

In any case, by the end of the last century, the exclusive practice of formal psychoanalysis had greatly declined. As the market shrunk, practitioners tended to offer therapy once a week, and/or to work in other domains of practice. Nonetheless, many aspects of psychoanalysis survive in other forms of therapy, using different terminology, even in methods (like CBT) that claim to be entirely unique. Again, research consistently supports the conclusion that all psychotherapies all work in much the same way, through understanding and validating feelings, and through teaching new ways of coping to patients (Wampold, 2001).

Unfortunately, psychoanalysis has not made the adjustments necessary to find a stable niche in 21st-century mental health systems. If one reads the most prominent journals devoted to psychoanalysis, it seems that little has changed over the decades. Here and there one sees formal research reports, but most articles continue to consist of theoretical speculations, supported only by case histories. This limited epistemology reflects the failure of psychoanalysis to establish affiliations with academic institutions.

This book will show how some psychoanalysts with research training have worked to build bridges to the scientific mainstream. I will refer to the work of research leaders in the previous generation, such as Lester Luborsky and Sidney Blatt, and to current leaders, such as Peter Fonagy.

I will review empirical data on aspects of psychoanalytic theory. I will show that by and large, while the classical theory has gained little support, new directions in research are being built, applying more evidence-based ideas, most particularly attachment theory.

I will examine the strength of empirical support for the effectiveness of psychoanalytic treatment. The book will show that there is good evidence for the efficacy of brief psychodynamic therapy, but little data to support the value of psychoanalysis lasting several years. (The only studies are pre-post comparisons, which lack control groups.) This suggests that most patients could be treated in a few months, and that extended courses of treatment can be reserved for patients who do not respond to short-term interventions.

The second part of the book concerns the boundaries of psychoanalysis. It will criticize the idea that the mental phenomena studied by psychoanalysis can, at this point, benefit from links to neuroscience (Panskepp and Solms, 2012). Psychological states can be studied in their own right, without recourse to trendy technologies. While imaging methods have made it possible to measure some of the neural correlates of thought, these relationships are specific. This is an example of a broader trend in modern psychology, in which neuroimaging has been commandeered to explain a very wide range of phenomena. This book will ask whether it is feasible to reduce complex mental constructs to specific neural mechanisms, many of which are still poorly understood.

The book will also examine the influence of psychoanalysis on the humanities. In recent decades, psychoanalytic theory has been fitted into post-modernist thought. I will briefly examine how the ideas of the maverick French psychoanalyst Jacques Lacan became central to that program (Roudinesco, 1990). But since these paradigms overtly reject empiricism, they take psychoanalysis further away from science.

Finally, this book will examine the social context of psychoanalysis, specifically how its ideas have created a "therapy culture" (Rieff, 1966; Furedi, 2004a, 2004b). These ideas favor nurture over nature, and tend to support the blaming of families for their children's problems. They also lead to what might be called the "psychologization" of the human condition, exemplified by the application of psychoanalytic ideas to history and biography.

This book will suggest that psychoanalytic thought could benefit from more humility. It is easy to come up with explanations for human problems, but they usually tell only one part of the story, and we are rarely in the position of being able to predict the future from the past.

A major theme of the book is that psychoanalysis needs to stop being isolated in its own institutes, and be integrated into the domain of clinical psychology. This principle suggests that its theory needs to become consistent with modern developmental psychology, and take gene-environment interactions into account. It also suggests that the practice of psychodynamic therapy needs to become an integrative and eclectic procedure that takes advantage of the best ideas from many schools of thought.

The future of psychoanalysis and its legacy

The world is better for the invention of psychoanalysis. Its ideas contain many grains of truth, and have left an important legacy to clinical psychology and psychiatry. Freud must be given credit for understanding that psychological interventions require an empathic relationship. Freud also promoted the understanding of life histories, and his followers have given a central role to empathy in psychotherapy. These principles have been supported by research, and remain essential for clinical work with patients.

This having been said, psychoanalysis must overcome its intellectual isolation and rejoin the mainstream of empiricism and science. Doing so will involve recognizing the contributions of other disciplines, whether or not they support traditional ideas. In this way, we can sidestep a dichotomous "yes-no" choice between psychoanalysis and opposition to psychoanalysis. Without exception, when a scientific paradigm is over a century old, it needs major revision. Psychoanalysis can accomplish this by giving up its splendid isolation, by finding a place in the mainstream of empirical research and evidence-based practice in psychology, and by offering treatment that is accessible and better integrated with other forms of psychotherapy.

References

Abbass, A.A., Kisely, S.R., Town, J.M., Leichsenring, F., Driessen, E., De Maat, S., Gerber, A., Dekker, J., Rabung, S., Rusalovska, S., Crowe, E.: Short-term psychodynamic psychotherapies for common mental disorders. *Cochrane Database of Systematic Reviews* 2014, (7). Art. No.: CD004687.

APA Presidential Task Force on Evidence-Based Practice: Evidence-based practice in psychology. *American Psychologist* 2006, 61: 271–285.

Bower, P., Gilboody, S.: Stepped care in psychological therapies: Access, effectiveness and efficiency. *British Journal of Psychiatry* 2005, 186: 11–17.

Eagle, M.N., Wolitsky, D.L.: Systematic empirical research versus clinical case studies: A valid antagonism? *Journal of the American Psychoanalytic Association* 2011, 69: 791–818.

Furedi, F.: *Therapy Culture: Cultivating Vulnerability in an Uncertain Age*. London, Routledge, 2004a.

Furedi, F.: *Paranoid Parenting*. London, Bloomsbury, 2004b.

Hale, N.: *The Rise and Crisis of Psychoanalysis in the United States*. New York, Oxford University Press, 1995.

Hoffman, I.Z.: Doublethinking our way to "scientific legitimacy": The desiccation of human experience. *Journal of the American Psychoanalytic Association* 2009, 57: 1043–1069.

Insel, T.R., Quirion, R.: Psychiatry as a clinical neuroscience discipline. *JAMA* 2005, 294: 2221–2224.

Lambert, M.J.: *Bergin and Garfield's Handbook of Psychotherapy and Behavior Change*. New York, Wiley, 2013.

Leichsenring, F., Rabung, S., Leibing, E.: The efficacy of short-term psychodynamic psychotherapy in specific psychiatric disorders: A meta-analysis. *Archives of General Psychiatry* 2004, 61: 1208–1216.

MacMillan, M.: *Freud Evaluated: The Completed Arc*. Cambridge, MA, MIT Press, 1991.

Panksepp, J, Solms, M. (2012) What is neuropsychoanalysis? Clinically relevant studies of the minded brain. Trends in Cognitive Science, 16: 6–8.

Roudinesco, E.: *Jacques Lacan & Co.: A History of Psychoanalysis in France, 1925–1985*. London, Free Association Books, 1990.

Sackett, D.L., Rosenberg, W.M., Gray, J.A., Haybes, R.B., Richardson, W.S.: Evidence based medicine: What it is and what it isn't. *BMJ* 1996, 312: 71–72.

Tamaskar, P., McGinnis, R.A.: Declining student interest in psychiatry. *JAMA* 2002, 287: 1859.

Vaillant, G.E.: Ego mechanisms of defense and personality psychopathology. *Journal of Abnormal Psychology* 1994, 103: 44–50.

Wampold, B.E.: *The Great Psychotherapy Debate: Models, Methods, and Findings*. Mahwah, NJ, Erlbaum Associates, 2001.

Part I

Psychoanalysis and science

Chapter 1

Psychoanalysis in decline

Psychoanalysis has had an enormous impact on clinical practice and modern culture. Yet over the last few decades of the century, its theory and practice have undergone a notable decline (Hale, 1995; Paris, 2005). Thirty years ago, it was already evident that analytic ideas were having much less impact on academic and clinical psychology (Westen, 1999). While these trends have long been in place, they have not been reversed. This is a dramatic change from the time when psychoanalysis was a strong leader in psychological science and mental health treatment (Paris, 2005).

In the US, while the total numbers of psychoanalysts in practice have not declined, psychiatrists are much less likely to become candidates in institutes, and the body of trainees is increasingly dominated by PhD psychologists. Candidates with a Master's level training in social work or nursing are also accepted. Moreover, candidates can enter training without degrees in *any* field related to mental health. The website of the American Psychoanalytic Association (www.apsa.org) mentions, among others, professions of educator, business consultant, historian, biographer, neuroscientist, and author. This is a major change from a time when most analysts had to have a medical degree. But opening up admission to institutes was necessary given major changes in who was willing to apply.

In my own field of psychiatry, there was a time when an analytic training was an important credential – one that was held by many chairs of university departments. Today department chairs tend to have a background in neuroscience. In the ten years (1997–2007) that I was chair of psychiatry at McGill University, and in the following decade, only one faculty member with training in psychoanalysis was hired on faculty, and there have been none since. (This is not because academic psychiatry discriminates against psychoanalysts, but because medical graduates are no longer inclined to seek this kind of training.)

The situation in psychology is in some ways even more discouraging for analysts. Even at the undergraduate level, abnormal psychology is no longer taught, as it once was, as a branch of psychoanalytic theory. And while psychodynamic approaches are still important for those who choose to be clinical psychologists, cognitive behavioral approaches are more prominent. Thus, although the large number of PhD graduates is enough to fill slots for analytic training, few of these programs encourage their graduates to become analysts or hire faculty who are likely to promote that option.

How can we explain the decline of a field whose ideas once dominated psychology, psychiatry, and related mental health disciplines? Several issues are in play. The first, related to a major theme of this book, is the intellectual isolation of a movement that trains prospective analysts in free-standing institutes that are not part of universities, and that do not encourage research (Kernberg, 2011, 2015). The guru-disciple relationship that tends to develop in a training analysis works against the adoption of scientific skepticism and a commitment to empiricism. A second issue is that psychoanalytic theory has had difficulty fitting its model into contemporary theory and research in psychology. That situation is not new (Fisher and Greenberg, 1996), but change has been very slow. A third issue is that psychoanalytic treatment, in its classical form, is expensive and relatively inaccessible.

Today, papers on psychoanalysis only occasionally appear in non-psychoanalytic journals, and research papers are rarely published in psychoanalytic journals. The pages of the two major journals in the field, the *International Journal of Psychoanalysis* and the *Journal of the American Psychoanalytic Association*, both sponsored by official psychoanalytic organizations, are almost entirely devoted to theoretical reviews, suggestions for practice, or case histories. *Psychoanalytic Psychology*, published by the American Psychological Association, does publish research, but its pages are still dominated by papers based on theory and/or case histories. *Psychoanalytic Inquiry*, published by Taylor and Francis, has shown interest in research, but most of its articles still lie outside the mainstream of psychology. The same can be said of the other journals related to psychoanalysis (*Psychoanalytic Quarterly*, *Psychoanalytic Review*, *Psychoanalytic Inquiry*, *American Journal of Psychoanalysis*, *Contemporary Psychoanalysis*, *Psychodynamic Psychiatry*, and the *Canadian Journal of Psychoanalysis*).

In retrospect, the isolation of psychoanalysis from other psychological disciplines was a serious error. The decision, originally made by Freud, was an understandable reaction to rejection of his ideas in academic circles. However, the dramatic rise of psychoanalysis in America (Hale, 1995) was a missed opportunity to develop a research culture. Today, with the important exception of attachment theory, little effort has been made to integrate psychodynamic theory into the paradigms that have become standard in developmental psychology. Psychoanalysis is also out of step with broader biosocial models, such as gene-environment interactions. As for practice, psychoanalytic therapy has played only a minor role in the psychotherapy integration movement.

Another trend is the move of medicine, psychiatry, and clinical psychology towards a commitment to evidence-based practice (Spring, 2007; Wallace, 2011). This trend implies that all treatments need to be validated by clinical trials, and further evaluated in meta-analyses. Practice should be based on what these data show. But since the time of Freud, psychoanalysis lacked a strong research tradition. Clinical experience is *not* a sufficient basis on which to offer complex and expensive forms of treatment.

A few psychoanalysts with PhD-level training in research methodology, such as the University of London professor Peter Fonagy (2015), have provided strong leadership in empirical investigation. Even so, as one can see from the content of journals, research remains outside the culture of analysis. This is one of the main reasons why the theory and practice of psychoanalysis, which have not been well supported by scientific evidence, need radical revision.

However, many of the formulations originally proposed by Freud have been quietly dropped. For this reason, the large literature of "Freud criticism" is not a useful way to examine the contemporary scene (Westen, 1999). Psychoanalysis in the 21st century has come to focus on concepts more strongly supported by research: understanding of the unconscious mind, and the relationship between life experiences and psychopathological symptoms.

A third issue in the decline of psychoanalysis is that the niche once assigned to psychoanalysis has been filled by competing methods, most particularly cognitive behavioral therapy (CBT; Beck, 1986). Moreover, CBT made great efforts, from the very beginning, to be evidence-based. CBT is the legacy of Aaron Beck (1986), a psychoanalyst who proposed this method as simpler, briefer, and researchable. Beck's commitment to science, leading to thousands of research studies, is largely responsible for the current reputation of CBT. Even so, CBT does not deserve its reputation as a method whose efficacy depends on the administration of specific technical interventions. As we will see, psychotherapies based on entirely different theories tend to produce very similar results (Wampold, 2001). But they have not all been studied as extensively as CBT. Actually, CBT does not come out as nearly as efficacious as it claims when the research literature is examined in detail (Wollfolk, 2010). But at least it has a tradition of respecting research findings from which psychoanalysis can learn.

A fourth problem concerns the length of treatment. When psychoanalysis was new, it was not that expensive, but it became more and more costly over time, particularly as the length of treatment increased. Today classical methods, with multiple weekly sessions over many months or years, are not affordable for all but a few of those who seek mental health treatment. This is an important reason why psychoanalytic treatment needs to be shortened and streamlined.

Research consistently shows that treatment with only a few months of psychodynamic therapy has a strong base in evidence (Leichsenring et al., 2004; Abbass et al., 2014). Recently, many people were surprised to learn that Pope Francis had seen a psychoanalyst in Argentina. But what the Pope described as analytic treatment was six months of once weekly sessions.

A fifth and closely related issue concerns the accessibility of treatment. Psychoanalysis continues to be practiced, mainly in large cities, but serves a small clientele who are willing to undergo a lengthy treatment. As documented decades ago in a book by the journalist Janet Malcolm (1981), practitioners, even in New York City, cannot easily make a living though psychoanalysis alone. In any case, psychoanalysis is not suitable for all patients. Here is how the website of the American Psychoanalytic Association (www.apsa.org/) describes who should seek this kind of treatment:

> The person best able to undergo psychoanalysis is someone who, no matter how incapacitated at the time, is basically, or potentially, a sturdy individual. This person may have already achieved important satisfactions – with friends, in marriage, in work, or through special interests and hobbies – but is nonetheless significantly impaired by long-standing symptoms: depression or anxiety, sexual incapacities, or physical symptoms without any demonstrable underlying physical

> cause. One person may be plagued by private rituals or compulsions or repetitive thoughts of which no one else is aware. Another may live a constricted life of isolation and loneliness, incapable of feeling close to anyone. A victim of childhood sexual abuse might suffer from an inability to trust others. Some people come to analysis because of repeated failures in work or in love, brought about not by chance but by self-destructive patterns of behavior. Others need analysis because the way they are – their character – substantially limits their choices and their pleasures. And still others seek analysis definitively to resolve psychological problems that were only temporarily or partially resolved by other approaches.

This description suggests that patients who are severely impaired are probably not suitable for analytic therapy, at least in its classical form. Instead, psychoanalysis seems to market itself for improving quality of life in people who are closer to normal than many of the patients seen in most clinics. Given the great demand for care for serious and disabling mental illness, this niche is too narrow, and helps account for the decline of the field. If a shortened and streamlined version of psychoanalysis is equally effective, the niche could be much wider.

Underlying all these problems, a sixth issue is the epistemological method of psychoanalysis. The use of case histories to support clinical theories runs a great danger of "confirmation bias", i.e., imposing previously held beliefs on the observation of phenomena (Sutherland, 2007). For this reason, clinical illustrations are no substitute for efficacy and effectiveness research on outcome, or for process research on the mechanisms behind therapeutic results. To put it another way, we now live in an era where accountability trumps authority. In an article on why clinical trials of psychoanalytic treatment are necessary, Eagle and Wolitsky (2012, p. 793) comment:

> For the most part, at least until recently, . . . calls for accountability and systematic research have gone unheeded. Although a smattering of psychoanalytic research was carried out over the years, only during the last two decades or so has there emerged a small but significant cadre of researchers who have focused on psychoanalysis and psychoanalytic treatment – virtually all of whom, it should be noted, are associated with universities rather than free-standing psychoanalytic

> institutes. However, neither the calls for research over the years nor the recent emergence of significant psychoanalytic research has had much impact on psychoanalytic training.

The most serious problem with relying on case histories is that they are, almost without exception, used to confirm conclusions rather than to disconfirm them. Great efforts always need to be made in science to keep confirmation biases out of research. Even in clinical trials, one can find "allegiance effects" in which investigators are more likely to report good outcome for the kind of therapy to which they already adhere (Luborsky et al., 1999).

In 2009 the *British Journal of Psychiatry* published a debate about whether the journal should accept psychoanalytic case reports (Wolpert and Fonagy, 2009). Wolpert, a biologist, argued that case reports should be excluded because they are not scientific. Fonagy, while conceding some of these points, defended analysis on the grounds that research is possible and is beginning to be conducted. But while Fonagy is strongly committed to science, he represents a small minority in a field which has notably lacked such a commitment. All too many analysts are still satisfied with papers that present theoretical arguments backed up by detailed reports about specific cases. Even worse, quite a few practitioners (e.g., Hoffman, 2009) see little need for research that fails to take a psychoanalytic perspective on clinical material.

In summary, the problem is that psychoanalysis has, up to recently, failed to build bridges with empirical sciences that could have provided it with needed intellectual fertilization. It has rejected reformulations of its theories that are based on data, so that had once been radical and new threatened to become conservative and stifling. A vast intellectual gulf between research and practice has emerged, in which psychoanalysts do no research, and in which its practitioners rarely read scientific journals that lie outside their field.

The problem goes back to Freud, who was satisfied with deriving theories from clinical inference. His attitude was not unusual at the time, as there was no such thing as evidence-based practice as we currently understand it. But standards are different today. Moreover, the philosopher Adolf Grunbaum (1984) noted that interpretations cannot be confirmed or validated simply by getting patients to agree with them. Clinicians' theories are strongly influenced by confirmation bias, and patients are often in a position of need that makes them likely to accept interpretations of any kind. For the clinician, the more strongly you believe in your own theory, the more likely you are to see what you observe as supporting it. This is why philosophers of science, such as Karl Popper (1968), have stated that psychoanalysis promoted ideas in ways constructed to resist all attempts at disproof.

Does psychoanalysis still have something important to offer, in spite of all these problems? For me the answer is a clear yes. While evidence-based practice should, at least in principle, be the norm, we need a psychodynamic perspective to do justice to the life histories of our patients. All too often, present-centered and symptom-centered models fail to take past histories sufficiently into account.

As a psychiatrist, I see my own discipline focusing on rebuilding bridges to the rest of medicine, adopting an almost purely biological model. Psychiatry now sees neuroscience, not psychology, as the basis of its practice. This narrowness of vision, and resultant loss of humanism, has been bad news for patients (Paris, 2017a). It is used to support a practice in which diagnoses are made by checklist, and drugs are prescribed for every symptom. Moreover, patients with psychological problems may receive narrowly based treatment using psychopharmacology, and may not necessarily be referred to competent practitioners of psychotherapy. Finally, when psychotherapy is offered, it should not consist only of non-specific support, but apply a broad armamentarium of interventions based on what research shows to be effective.

Freud criticism

In the last 20 years, some of the most influential criticisms of psychoanalysis have come from outside the scientific and clinical communities. Unfortunately, most of these critics have focused on Freud's original ideas, with a lack of informed comment about the many ways in which contemporary psychoanalysis has evolved over the years.

A group of Freud scholars, most trained in the humanities or philosophy, led this project. Frederick Crews, professor of English literature at the University of California, Berkeley, is probably the best known, and followed a series of articles in *The New York Review of Books* with a recent book-length critique (Crews, 2017).

Crews had taught psychoanalytic criticism of literature to his students, but came to disbelieve the theory after concluding that it could be used to prove almost anything. More generally, Crews emphasized that Freud's clinical methods imposed a predetermined structure, and failed to test hypotheses in a way that others could replicate. He saw the analytic method as more reminiscent of indoctrination than of open-minded inquiry. His recent book argued that psychoanalysis was a personal cause for Freud, and was never designed to be tested scientifically.

The psychoanalytic movement has resisted this kind of criticism, often dismissing it as "Freud-bashing". Needless to say, one should never judge the value of ideas on the basis of the personal failings of an author. And Crews seems to be unaware of how much the field has changed since Freud's time. However, if psychoanalysis wants to join the scientific community, its critics need to be taken seriously.

When Freud and psychoanalysis fall under attack, the discipline can readily find defenders. In a culture where so many prominent intellectuals had spent years being analyzed themselves, there has been no lack of advocates. A good example was the political scientist Paul Roazen, whose unusual career has been described by his former student, Todd Dufresne (2007). (Dufresne, a philosophy professor, is a prominent practitioner of Freud criticism.) Roazen was trained as a political scientist, but spent his life studying psychoanalysis. In the 1970s, he moved to Toronto and came to prominence as a Freud critic. Roazen (1975) showed the extent to which the analytic movement had been influenced by power struggles, and how Freud had used his own power in questionable ways. He was the first author to document that Freud had psychoanalyzed his own daughter Anna.

Yet as Roazen grew older, he stated he was tired of being a heretic, and became a passionate defender of Freud, one who could be counted on to carry out counter-attacks on critics. Shortly before his death, I became Roazen's target when, in spite of his negative comments in peer review for the publisher, the University of Toronto Press published my book (Paris, 2005) about the loss of influence of psychoanalysis in academic psychiatry.

Freud criticism is somewhat misdirected, in that it is historical, and has not given sufficient emphasis to contemporary developments. Neither the critics nor the defenders of Freud have properly addressed whether well-designed scientific research supports contemporary theory and practice. Again, one need not embrace ideas that were current a hundred years ago to find continued value in psychodynamic ideas. In any case, these criticisms, however justified, have had more impact on humanists and intellectuals than on scientists, many of whom have long dismissed Freud because of the absence of empirical data to justify his conclusions.

How psychoanalysis failed to adopt a research culture

After the 1960s, the dominance of psychoanalysis was about to come to an end. Few of us anticipated this development. Young psychiatrists like me were fascinated with psychoanalytic theory, because it seemed to plumb the deepest and most mysterious aspects of the human mind. Its insights were clinical, and seemed too subtle to be operationalized for research.

Yet at much the same time, psychiatry wanted to rejoin medicine, and clinical psychology became interested in other methods of therapy. Psychiatry already had a robust tradition of biological research and practice, and clinicians routinely used antipsychotic and antidepressant drugs for conditions that might previously have been treated with talking therapy alone. Over the next few decades, managing mental illness with drugs became almost entirely dominant among physicians.

Ironically, at the very same time, research on psychotherapy was taking off. This development was stimulated by criticism – in a famous paper, the British psychologist Hans Eysenck (1952) argued that improvement in symptoms under then-standard psychotherapy did not exceed rates of naturalistic remission. This led to a large body of research by academic psychologists using modern methods of evaluating evidence, particularly the randomized controlled trials that are standard in clinical pharmacology. This research refuted Eysenck, showing that on the whole, psychotherapy is usually efficacious for most of the problems that patients bring to clinics (Smith et al., 1980; Lambert, 2013). But it did not support the practice of psychoanalysis.

Moreover, only a few members of the larger psychoanalytic community and its supporters (Strupp, 1971; Luborsky and Luborsky, 2006; Blatt et al., 2007; Westen, 1999) became seriously involved in psychotherapy research. On a practical level, as long as analytic treatment was lengthy rather than brief, investigations of classical psychoanalysis would be costly. But there was a deeper problem: training in psychoanalysis had never encouraged empirical investigation, and the theoretical papers required for those who want to become training analysts are almost always theoretical (Kernberg, 2000). Younger practitioners have lacked role models to conduct research.

Instead, most psychoanalysts have considered that their clinical methods provide insights into the mind that could not be accessed in any other way. They see their approach as the best way to access the unconscious mind. And since many who practice this kind of therapy are good with words, they are also good at convincing others that their views are valid. In my experience directing residency training programs in psychiatry, analysts are still greatly admired for their teaching, and their sense of certainty remains appealing to many trainees.

Moreover, in spite of the commonalities between psychoanalysis and other forms of psychotherapy, its practitioners have not always been open to other points of view. When I applied in my final year of training for a position at a student mental health clinic that specialized in psychotherapy, the analyst who interviewed me asked what my theoretical position was. I said I was interested in psychoanalysis, but wanted to take other models into account. His reply was: "and just what might these others be?" I can also remember hearing the analyst Peter Sifneos presenting at a conference: when challenged to present evidence for his views about the Oedipus complex, he defended his commitment by simply stating: "I am a psychoanalyst".

I have to wonder whether such a strong adherence to one method has been affected by the fact that practitioners are required to undergo their own analysis. Perhaps they are hesitant to be ungrateful and to rebel against the senior clinicians who provided them with personal guidance.

Another problem is that psychoanalysis is resource-intensive and available only to a minority of potential patients. More people should be able to benefit from psychological treatment. From early in my career, I have been interested in making psychotherapy accessible. My hope has been to adapt the principles of psychoanalysis and other forms of talking therapy in a more practical form. I also wanted to treat more patients, which meant I have seen most of them more briefly. Psychoanalysis is a treatment that lasts for years, and even if it were insured, it would have a long waiting list. I saw this happen in 1970, when psychiatrists in Canada were insured by a single governmental payer for all their work; the result was that they quickly filled up their practices, and had to turn down all further referrals, recreating the shortage that universal insurance had aimed to redress.

Yet in the 1970s, many clinicians became interested in short-term, time-limited psychotherapy that lasts for a few months (Garfield, 1998). After a large conference on these methods was held in Montreal in 1976, clinics offering this kind of therapy were set up at several teaching hospitals. (Even so, senior analysts muttered about the impossibility of helping patients within a few months.) Yet today the best evidence for the efficacy of any psychological treatment lies in brief therapy, whether it is psychodynamic in orientation, or cognitive behavioral (Lambert, 2013). Research shows that many patients can be successfully managed in brief treatment (Leichsenring et al., 2004), for which most people are either insured, or can directly afford.

Forty years ago, evidence-based practice was still in its infancy. Students still tended to defer to the clinical experience of their teachers. In medical schools, practice was almost always driven by expert consensus rather than hard facts. When a senior professor expressed an opinion, nobody was likely to challenge him by saying: "show me your data". Medicine was as much an art as a science, and psychiatry was particularly far from being empirically grounded.

Moreover, as a young clinician, I was impressed by the therapeutic triumphs of biological psychiatry. I saw how drugs were transforming the treatment of severe mental disorders. A state hospital I visited as an undergraduate in the 1950s had 4,000 beds, but after the introduction of effective drugs, eventually closed entirely. As a resident in psychiatry, I was the first physician at my training site to prescribe lithium to control mania. (The patient went on to make a miraculous recovery.) I also saw good results with antidepressants, even though I gradually came to see their limitations (Paris, 2010).

Yet when it came to psychotherapy, I could see no intellectual or practical alternative to the use of psychodynamic models. In the first half of my career, I was viewed as a supporter of psychoanalysis. I found behavior therapy to be mechanical, based on a theory that ignored mental processes considered as a "black box" not open to measurement. I remember one psychology student insisting that one could not speak of patients hearing voices, but only of their reporting such experiences. These problems were largely overcome when behavior therapy was replaced by modern cognitive behavioral therapy.

Living in a culture that took psychoanalytic ideas for granted, I was in the same position as people in previous centuries surrounded by a culture of religious belief. It was unthinkable to reject a dominant paradigm. Psychoanalysis, and only psychoanalysis, took the issues that led me to become a psychiatrist seriously. Its ideas were not only applicable to mental illness, but to the human condition. Psychodynamics made psychiatry into a field that dealt with life itself. Moreover, I could not see how insights into the mind drawn from clinical encounters could ever be scientifically tested, or how such complex problems could even be studied.

What I failed to see was that scientific medicine and psychological research could evolve new methods to shed light on these questions. In the end, empirical findings derived from these approaches would lead to different conclusions. Given my medical training, and an undergraduate degree in psychology, I should have understood that the evaluation of any treatment must be guided by scientific principles.

The problem with classical psychoanalysis was that it did not generate hypotheses that could be put to the test. Instead, like a religion, it idealized its founder, and re-interpreted his good ideas, while failing to discard the bad ones. Psychoanalysis failed to build bridges with empirical sciences that could have provided it with needed intellectual fertilization and provide renewal. It rejected reformulations of its theories, and some of the most fruitful revisions were, at least initially, treated as heresy. This led to the vast intellectual gulf between research and practice, in which psychoanalysts hardly ever read scientific journals and did not encourage empirical investigation.

The claim that the clinical method used by most analysts is scientific (Wallerstein, 2009) reflects a failure to understand how science works. Clinicians' theories can be idiosyncratic and influenced by multiple cognitive biases. The more strongly therapists believe in their theory, the more likely they are to interpret everything they observe as confirming it.

Moreover, as academic psychiatry tried to become a medical specialty like any other, younger psychiatrists were no longer attracted to psychoanalysis, and some who had joined the movement eventually left it to espouse other models (Paris, 2005). It took me many years to go through my own transition. But I eventually came to treat patients with an integrated eclectic model that drew on ideas from many schools of psychotherapy. This point of view is particularly necessary in the population I work with: patients who suffer from borderline personality disorder (Paris, 2017b). I had learned a great deal from psychoanalysis, but developed a commitment to empirical science, and began a second career in research on personality disorders.

Today, while psychoanalysis in its original form is still practiced, most patients are offered an adaptation: *psychodynamic psychotherapy*, in which patients sit up instead of lying on a couch, and are seen once a week, or *brief psychodynamic therapy*, in which patients are seen weekly for a few months (Gabbard, 2014). In any case, the market for therapy three to four times a week is no longer there. One survey (Cherry et al., 2004) found that most of the graduates of an analytic institute were not practicing classical psychoanalysis, but seeing most of their patients once a week.

But there are now hundreds of forms of psychotherapy, some of which are derivatives of Freud's ideas and procedures, while others are variations of CBT. Unfortunately, all too many therapies are trendy ideas promoting methods that have not been researched to find out how well they work. Instead, therapies are usually promoted through books, conferences, and workshops.

Today the field of psychological treatment is dominated by CBT, the method that has had the strongest evidence base. On the surface, CBT does not seem to resemble psychoanalysis. It focuses on changing the way people think in the present, and pays less attention to childhood experiences. Yet CBT was the brain-child of a trained psychoanalyst. It even has a construct to describe the impact of early experience – cognitive *schemas*. Beck, unlike his former colleagues, subjected his treatment method to clinical trials and showed that it usually worked within a manageable period of time. The movement to evidence-based practice helps explain the striking success of CBT.

Meanwhile, psychoanalysis continued to be resistant to scientific investigation of its ideas. This went against the spirit of the times in both psychiatry and psychology. An article by an analyst who also conducts research, entitled "The Impending Death of Psychoanalysis" (Bornstein, 2001), pointed out how a lack of commitment to empiricism contributed to a striking decline in the influence of psychoanalysis.

Even so, important voices within the psychoanalytic movement have promoted research. The British psychoanalyst-researcher Peter Fonagy, a major figure in personality disorder research, has been consistent in his advocacy. Otto Kernberg has often collaborated with researchers, and published an important paper on the results of psychoanalytic treatment at the Menninger Clinic (Kernberg, 1973). He also helped develop an evidence-based form of psychodynamic therapy for borderline personality disorder (Yeomans et al., 2015).

Another voice in favor of science comes from two psychoanalyst-researchers, Robert Bornstein and Steven Huprich, who edited a special issue of the journal *Psychoanalytic Inquiry*. Consider the following passage from their article (2015, p. 186):

> A curious dissociation characterizes contemporary clinical psychology and psychiatry. On the one hand, Freud remains the most widely cited author in psychology journal articles (with 13,900 citations overall during the five-year period surveyed). These data suggest Freud's continuing influence, but consider: The number of clinical psychologists who describe themselves as psychoanalytic declined from 36% in 1960 to 18% in 1997, and fewer than 5% of doctoral programs in clinical psychology now describe themselves as emphasizing psychodynamic approaches. Citations of psychoanalytic literature have declined, and less than 1% of doctoral dissertations contain keywords related to psychoanalysis.
>
> The insularity of the psychoanalytic community has been a primary cause of the decline of psychoanalysis during the past several decades. Having little interest in empirical data, many analysts make untested claims based on little more than anecdotal clinical evidence – evidence obtained behind closed doors, in the privacy of the consulting room. Oftentimes these assertions conflict with well-established findings in clinical, social, developmental, and cognitive psychology.

If the views of analysts like Bornstein and Huprich held more sway, one might not even have to talk about the decline of psychoanalysis. Similar views have been published by other writers who describe the problem as "bridging the great divide" (Chiesa, 2010). As Bornstein (2005, p. 325) put it in another article:

> the diminished influence of contemporary psychoanalysis is largely a product of theory mismanagement: Rather than looking forward (to the evolving demands of science and practice) and outward (to ideas and findings in other areas of psychology and medicine), many psychoanalysts have chosen to look backward (at the seminal but dated contributions of early psychoanalytic practitioners) and inward (at their like-minded colleagues' own analytic writings). As a result, psychoanalysts committed seven "deadly sins" that exacerbated the theory's decline: insularity, inaccuracy, indifference, irrelevance, inefficiency, indeterminacy, and insolence.

Instead of entering a new era in which analysis joins with and contributes to psychological science, too many practitioners continue to believe that their method allows for an "in-depth" view of the mind that no empirical study can access. But those who refuse to accept the rules of science will inevitably be cast out of its temple.

Summary

The decline of psychoanalysis is related to many factors. First, it has become intellectually isolated from other disciplines, creating what political commentators sometimes call an "echo chamber". Second, it has failed to make a strong commitment to the principles of evidence-based practice. Third, it has failed to encourage integration with other methods of psychotherapy. Fourth, the treatment is costly and inaccessible. Fifth, its method of clinical inference fails to meet the standards of empirical science.

References

Abbass, A.A., Kisely, S.R., Town, J.M., Leichsenring, F., Driessen, E., De Maat, S., Gerber, A., Dekker, J., Rabung, S., Rusalovska, S., Crowe, E.: Short-term psychodynamic psychotherapies for common mental disorders. *Cochrane Database of Systematic Reviews* 2014, (7). Art. No.: CD004687.

Beck, A.T.: *Cognitive Therapy and the Emotional Disorders*. New York, Basic Books, 1986.

Blatt, S.J., Besser, A., Ford, R.Q.: Two primary configurations of psychopathology and change in thought disorder in long-term, intensive, inpatient treatment of seriously disturbed young adults. *American Journal of Psychiatry* 2007, 164: 1561–1567.

Bornstein, R.F.: The impending death of psychoanalysis. *Psychoanalytic Psychology* 2001, 18: 3–20.

Bornstein, R.F.: Reconnecting psychoanalysis to mainstream psychology: Challenges and opportunities. *Psychoanalytic Psychology* 2005, 22: 323–340.

Bornstein, R.F., Huprich, S.K.: Behind closed doors: Sadomasochistic enactments and psychoanalytic research. *Psychoanalytic Inquiry* 2015, 35, suppl 1: 185–195.

Cherry, S., Cabaniss, D.L., Forand, N.R., Roose, S.P.: Psychoanalytic practice in the early postgraduate years. *Journal of the American Psychoanalytic Association* 2004, 52: 851–871.

Chiesa, M.: Research and psychoanalysis: Still time to bridge the great divide? *Psychoanalytic Psychology* 2010, 27: 99–114.

Crews, F.: *Freud: The Making of an Illusion*. New York, Henry Holt, 2017.

Dufresne, T.: *Against Freud, the Critics Talk Back*. Stanford, CA, Stanford University Press, 2007.

Eagle, M.N., Wolitsky, D.L.: Systematic empirical research versus clinical case studies: A valid antagonism? *Journal of the American Psychoanalytic Association* 2012, 69: 791–818.

Eysenck, H.: The effects of psychotherapy: An evaluation. *Journal of Consulting Psychology* 1952, 16: 319–324.

Fisher, S., Greenberg, R.P.: *Freud Scientifically Reappraised.* New York, Wiley, 1996.

Fonagy, P.: The effectiveness of psychodynamic psychotherapies: An update. *World Psychiatry* 2015, 14: 1137–1150.

Gabbard, G.O.: *Psychodynamic Psychiatry in Clinical Practice*, 5th edition. Washington, DC, American Psychiatric Publishing, 2014.

Garfield, S.L.: *The Practice of Brief Psychotherapy.* New York, Wiley, 1998.

Grunbaum, A.: *The Foundations of Psychoanalysis.* Berkeley, CA, University of California Press, 1984.

Hale, N.: *The Rise and Crisis of Psychoanalysis in the United States.* New York, Oxford University Press, 1995.

Hoffman, I.Z.: Doublethinking our way to "scientific legitimacy": The desiccation of human experience. *Journal of the American Psychoanalytic Association* 2009, 57: 1043–1069.

Kernberg, O.F.: Summary and conclusions of Psychotherapy and psychoanalysis, final report of the Menninger Foundation's Psychotherapy Research Project. *International Journal of Psychiatry* 1973, 11: 62–77.

Kernberg, O.F.: A concerned critique of psychoanalytic education. *International Journal of Psycho-Analysis* 2000, 81: 97–104.

Kernberg, O.F.: Psychoanalysis and the university: A difficult relationship. *International Journal of Psycho-Analysis* 2011, 92: 609–622.

Kernberg, O.F.: Resistances and progress in developing a research framework in psychoanalytic institutes. *Psychoanalytic Inquiry* 2015, 35, suppl 1: 98–114.

Lambert, M.J.: *Bergin and Garfield's Handbook of Psychotherapy and Behavior Change*, 6th edition. New York, Wiley, 2013.

Leichsenring, F., Rabung, S., Leibing, E.: The efficacy of short-term psychodynamic psychotherapy in specific psychiatric disorders: A meta-analysis. *Archives of General Psychiatry* 2004, 61: 1208–1216.

Luborsky, L., Diguer, L., Seligman, D.A., Rosenthal, R., Krause, E.D., Johnson, S.: The researcher's own therapy allegiances: A "wild card" in comparisons of treatment efficacy. *Clinical Psychology: Science and Practice* 1999, 6: 95–106.

Luborsky, L., Luborsky, E.: *Research and Psychotherapy: The Vital Link.* Lanham, MD, Rowman & Littlefield, 2006.

Malcolm, J.: *Psychoanalysis: The Impossible Profession.* New York, Knopf, 1981.

Paris, J.: *The Fall of an Icon: Psychoanalysis and Academic Psychiatry.* Toronto, University of Toronto Press, 2005.

Paris, J.: *The Use and Misuse of Psychiatric Drugs: An Evidence-Based Guide.* London, John Wiley, 2010.

Paris, J.: *Psychotherapy in an Age of Neuroscience.* New York, Oxford University Press, 2017a.

Paris, J.: *Stepped Care for Borderline Personality Disorder: Making Treatment Brief, Effective, and Accessible.* New York, Academic Press/Elsevier, 2017b.

Popper, K.: *Conjectures and Refutations.* New York, Harper Torch, 1968.

Roazen, P.: *Freud and His Followers.* New York, Knopf, 1975.

Smith, M.L., Glass, G.V., Miller, T.: *The Benefits of Psychotherapy.* Baltimore, Johns Hopkins Press, 1980.

Spring, B.: Evidence-based practice in clinical psychology: What it is, why it matters: What you need to know. *Journal of Clinical Psychology* 2007: 611–631.
Strupp, H.H.: *Psychotherapy and the Modification of Abnormal Behavior: An Introduction to Theory and Research*. New York, McGraw Hill, 1971.
Sutherland, S.: *Irrationality*, 2nd edition. London, Pinter and Martin, 2007.
Wallace, J.: The practice of evidence-based psychiatry today. *Advances in Psychiatric Treatment* 2011, 17: 389–395.
Wallerstein, R.S.: What kind of research in psychoanalytic science? *International Journal of Psychoanalysis* 2009, 90: 109–133.
Wampold, B.E.: *The Great Psychotherapy Debate: Models, Methods, and Findings*. Mahwah, NJ, Erlbaum Associates, 2001.
Westen, D.: The scientific status of unconscious processes: Is Freud really dead? *Journal of the American Psychoanalytic Association*1999, 47: 1061–1106.
Wollfolk, R.L.: *The Value of Psychotherapy: The Talking Cure in an Age of Clinical Science*. New York, Guilford Press, 2010.
Wolpert, L., Fonagy, P.: There is no place for the psychoanalytic case report in the British Journal of Psychiatry. *British Journal of Psychiatry* 2009, 195: 483–487.
Yeomans, F., Clarkin, J.F., Kernberg, O.F.: *Transference-Focused Psychotherapy for Borderline Personality Disorder: A Clinical Guide*. Washington, DC, American Psychiatric Publishing, 2015.

Chapter 2

Reconciling psychoanalysis and research

Is it possible to reconcile psychoanalysis with contemporary scientific research in psychology? Again, contemporary psychoanalysis should not be judged by the version promoted during Freud's lifetime. Many changes have occurred since then, as older ideas were quietly dropped and replaced by new ones (Fonagy, 2015). As Westen (1998, p. 333) commented:

> Psychodynamic theory and therapy have evolved considerably since 1939 when Freud's bearded countenance was last sighted in earnest. Contemporary psychoanalysts and psychodynamic therapists no longer write much about ids and egos, nor do they conceive of treatment for psychological disorders as an archaeological expedition in search of lost memories . . . psychotherapists who rely on theories derived from Freud do not typically spend their time lying in wait for phallic symbols. They pay attention to sexuality, because it is an important part of human life and intimate relationships and one that is often filled with conflict. Today, however, most psychodynamic theorists and therapists spend much of their time helping people with problematic interpersonal patterns, such as difficulty getting emotionally intimate or repeatedly getting intimate with the wrong kind of person.

Nonetheless, while retaining a focus on contemporary psychoanalysis, let us review how much support some of the crucial ideas associated with psychoanalysis have gained from research. I will not go into great detail in examining this literature, since previous publications have dealt with these issues in detail. Almost all authors have come to the conclusion that some of Freud's ideas need to be discarded, and that analysis needs to revise those that can be retained (Fisher and Greenberg, 1996; Eagle, 2011).

The unconscious mind

The concept of an unconscious mind was Freud's most important contribution to psychology. Historians, such as Henri Ellenberger (1970), have pointed out that Freud was not the first person to describe the unconscious, given that one can find 19th-century thinkers with similar ideas. But every innovation has its predecessors. Freud was the first to suggest that unconscious processes are a factor in the development of mental disorders. But the mechanisms of the unconscious mind are more indirect and complex than he imagined. The idea that most mental activity is unconscious is crucial, but we are just beginning to understand the relationship between emotion and reasoned thought.

There has long been empirical evidence that many if not most mental processes lie outside conscious awareness (Kihlstrom, 1987), and recent research has strengthened the same conclusion (Kihlstrom, 2015). But this is not the sort of unconscious that Freud postulated. We now understand that most brain functions are carried out without conscious thought, i.e., there is a *cognitive unconscious*, in which many aspects of perception, motor skills, and memory are automatized or stored outside of awareness. This concept describes the way the brain carries out tasks without the delays associated with reasoning out every decision.

In the past some psychologists (and many economists) have mistakenly assumed that people primarily use thought to reach rational decisions. But as the Scottish Philosopher David Hume (1739/1882) famously put it: "reason is a slave to the passions". Research in cognitive science has shown that thoughts are always based on feelings (Damasio, 2005). There is also strong evidence that emotions can be unconscious (Westen, 1998; Bargh, 2017). Research in behavioral economics comes to a similar overall conclusion: that emotions tend to trump rationality (Thaler, 2015; Kahnemann, 2011).

Current methods of measuring unconscious process in research are much more sophisticated than the clinical observations that Freud relied on. For example, one can study these phenomena by using cuing and association of words (Bargh, 2017), or by subliminal stimuli (Bornstein and Masling, 1998; Dehaene, 2014).

By and large, Freud's image of the mind as an iceberg, most of which is submerged, has been supported. On the other hand, research has not supported his concept that the unconscious mind is largely ruled by hidden drives and desires, or that the role of the conscious mind is to repress these urges. A better way to think about this relationship is that many mental processes need to be automatic, while the conscious mind is most responsible for decision-making that takes time and careful consideration.

Memory

There is a very large literature describing research on human memory (Schachter, 2008). In the light of these findings, Freud's ideas require radical revision. The hypothesis that memory is a kind of videotape, recording all life events in detail turns out to be incorrect and impossible – even given the large capacity of the brain for the storage of experience. Natural selection has produced an efficient brain, using a memory system that is selective, and that does not permanently record all data (Lane et al., 2015). Since the brain's "hard drive" has limited space, we need to forget most things that happen to us. (Perhaps that is fortunate.) It has also been difficult to establish whether memories of past events can either be "repressed" or accurately recovered; on the other hand, false memories can be easily implanted by contexts and suggestions (Loftus and Ketcham, 1994).

The idea that early childhood memories are lost because they become unconscious is also incorrect. The reason we do not remember childhood events is that the brain is immature at that stage of life, and does not have the capacity to make permanent records of experience (Schachter, 1995). Hardly anyone can remember events before age two, and few memories before age five remain available to adults.

Most importantly, research shows that memory is *reconstructive*, and is not an accurate image of past events (Lane et al., 2015). Each time we access a memory, the details of past events are remembered differently, so that traces of the past are influenced by more recent life events. Contrary to Freud's theory, memories are selectively retained, and many are either lost or greatly modified. In spite of great effort, research has not been able to confirm the phenomenon of repression as originally hypothesized by Freud (Bower, 1990; Loftus and Ketcham, 1994).

For all these reasons, memories of childhood are not necessarily an accurate recording of the past. What we seem to remember is a *narrative* that tells a story, but is factually unreliable. And given that memory is a reconstruction in the light of later events, some of the childhood traumas suggested to patients by therapists may never have happened, even when they offer a narrative that seems to explain so much. (Chapter 9 will show how an overly literal belief in Freud's theory of repression led to the great scandal of the "recovered memory" movement of the 1990s.) Modern research on memory has taken the unconscious into account by describing differences between *explicit* and *implicit* memory (Schacter, 1995). But it does not follow that repression is the *usual* reason why life experiences are not remembered. Like a computer that has limited storage, the brain maintains efficiency by discarding old data.

Childhood determinism

The idea that childhood shapes adult personality and mental symptoms has had a great influence on how educated people think about human nature, and how therapists think about their patients. The grain of truth in these ideas is that early experience can have lasting effects, and that life histories are important. However, the theory requires serious revision. Early experiences, particularly when cumulative and negative, can be risk factors for later problems. But childhood does not strictly determine adult psychopathology. I reviewed this literature in a previous book (Paris, 2000), leading to the conclusion that the impact of childhood experiences can only be understood in interaction with temperamental factors that vary between one person and another.

The psychological development of children is much more complex than Freud believed. The psychosexual stages he posited have not been supported by empirical evidence (Fisher and Greenberg, 1996). Erikson's (1950) reformulation of these stages in a psychosocial context may have had more clinical relevance, but it also failed to obtain consistent research support (Rutter and Rutter, 1993). As for the claim that resolving an Oedipus complex is crucial for psychological development, this central pillar of Freud's thought is rarely invoked today. As Eagle (2017, p. 294) comments:

> I know of no body of research evidence supporting the iconic psychoanalytic hypothesis that the way in which the individual resolves the Oedipus complex is a significant factor in the development of psychopathology or in central psychological areas in an individual's life such as the formation of gender identity or the development of conscience.

Meanwhile, developmental psychology has moved in a very different direction. There are large individual differences in the effects of adversity, and research supports a crucial role for interactions between temperament and experience (Kagan, 2006). Since people differ genetically in their personality traits, some respond to negative life events more than others (Fonagy, 2003; Belsky and Pluess, 2009).

The more general idea that early childhood experience, particularly when it involves severe adversities, can shape adult personality and psychopathology has a degree of empirical support. But there is no one-to-one correspondence between any early life event and adult outcome. The work of the British child psychiatrist, Michael Rutter, has been crucial for understanding these complex relationships (Rutter and Rutter, 1993). He was involved with a well-known study of Romanian orphans, supported by findings from several other countries, showing that infants receiving minimum care for extended periods had deficits in development that remained apparent many years later (Woodhouse et al., 2017).

This having been said, extreme examples do not necessarily support the idea that infancy or early childhood must *always* be more important than later life events. For one thing, problems that start early in life tend to continue over time. The relationship between childhood and adulthood is more complex and multivariate than Freud ever imagined. Moreover, the idea that what happens in the first few years of life is crucial ignores the role of other factors that are much more predictive of adult outcome, such as social class (Kagan, 1998).

Thus, one cannot assume that a specific childhood event will produce predictable consequences, or that every specific adult problem has sources in early development. To understand this relationship, one needs to consider temperamental variations, as well as the role of resilience (Rutter, 2012a). Individual variations in sensitivity to the environment are an area that psychoanalytic theories have failed to address.

The long-term impact of childhood events is governed not by the nature of experience alone, but by gene-environment interactions (Rutter, 2012b). Thus, genetic factors determine the extent to which people are sensitive or insensitive to their environment, and high sensitivity can lead to either positive or negative responses to life events (Belsky and Pluess, 2009).

Moreover, single traumatic events do not, by themselves, lead to psychopathology, but are mediated by a large series of experiences over the life span (Rutter and Rutter, 1993). For all these reasons, one cannot explain mental disorders as *primarily* due to traumatic experiences in the past. Adverse events in early development are certainly a risk factor for many mental disorders. But we need to invoke a model in which childhood experience is one of several interacting variables that increase the risk for psychopathology.

Childhood trauma is a subject that arouses strong emotions, both among clinicians and in the general public. But research in community populations shows that most people who experience early trauma grow up to function reasonably well in life, and that most people who suffer adversity in childhood will not develop mental disorders (Rutter, 2012b). Risks are also dose-dependent; if traumatic experiences are subtle and difficult to identify, they may not have played a large role. Thus, the effects of childhood experience, whether traumatic or emotionally neglectful, are important factors in development, but do not, as once thought, firmly determine personality or psychological symptoms later in life. Resilience is not the exception, but the rule.

Another important line of research that illuminates this issue is *behavior genetics*, a field of psychology that measures the heritability of traits by comparing concordance in identical vs. fraternal twins (Jang, 2008). Using this method, one can show that genes shape about half the variance affecting any adult trait or symptom. Strikingly, when one compares personality characteristics in children raised in the same family, they are no more similar than perfect strangers. Again, this is not to say that childhood experience plays *no* role in psychological development. But its long-term impact depends on interactions with inborn traits and the social environment (as well as a good degree of luck).

These findings contradict the theory of childhood determinism. Adverse experiences in childhood are *risk factors*, but not direct causes of psychopathology. In other words, they increase the statistical likelihood of mental illness, but mainly affect those who are already vulnerable in some way. This helps explain why early trauma, by itself, does not consistently lead to symptoms later in life. Mental disorders do not develop unless early adversities are combined with inborn predispositions and later adversities.

Psychoanalysis has had a profound influence on how people think about child development and parenting. (Chapter 8 will examine how the fear of traumatizing one's own children has become a major theme of "therapy culture".) Many therapists influenced by psychoanalysis have made the mistake of generalizing observations drawn from clinical experience and turning them into scientific "laws" to predict outcomes. Since clinicians derive conclusions from work with symptomatic patients, they may not be aware of the ubiquity of resilience in those who have suffered adversity, or that many people with mental illnesses have never experienced traumatic childhoods. It therefore makes little sense, as psychoanalysts sometimes do, to spend years trying to unearth early life events to explain current life problems.

While it is tempting to believe that childhood adversity explains adult psychopathology, for every person we see with a traumatic history, many others never have symptoms or come to clinical attention. The term *resilience* (Rutter, 2012b) refers to the ability to "bounce back" from the impact of adverse events. We can think of it as a defense system against psychological injury. Just as immunological mechanisms protect us against the physical attack of micro-organisms, resilience mechanisms protect us against the emotional effects of adverse events. Resilience, like any other capacity, varies greatly between individuals. It depends on capacities intrinsic to the individual, characteristics rooted in temperament. This is why most people with traumatic childhoods do not develop diagnosable mental disorders or come for treatment.

Another way to understand these relationships is that the way that experiences affect us depends on how the mind assimilates them (Plomin et al., 2012). Personality traits, rooted in temperament, are mechanisms designed to deal with a variety of challenges from the environment. They play a crucial role in determining how any life event, whether negative or positive, is processed in our minds. These gene-environment (or person-environment) interactions are stronger predictors of outcome than exposure to adversity alone.

Children who carry predispositions to mental disorders, or who have temperamental vulnerabilities that make them unusually sensitive to stress, are more likely to experience adverse life events as negative, and to react badly to them (Ellis et al., 2011). In contrast, children with positive personality traits tend to find ways to cope with adversity, making them relatively immune to stressful experiences. Although most children lie on a continuum between these extremes, an average child will have sufficient resourcefulness to weather an average level of adversity. This is why the theory of "differential susceptibility" to the environment (Belsky and Pluess, 2009) has both evolutionary and neurodevelopmental significance. Thus, research shows that those who are most sensitive to adverse events will also benefit more from positive events. If stressors are both severe and multiple, then damage is more likely. By and large, children are generally much tougher and more flexible than many people think. It is better to have a happy childhood than an unhappy one, but statistical associations are not strong enough for prediction of the future.

Another conclusion is that trauma is more pathogenic when it is multiple and cumulative (Rutter, 2012b). Important adverse events during childhood, such as family discord, parental psychopathology, and poor socioeconomic status, are inter-correlated and lead to cumulative effects. In summary, when risks pile up, they are more likely to continue to affect development into adolescence and young adulthood. But the search for a single traumatic event, an idea that has influenced the thinking of many therapists, is a simplification that is contradicted by a large body of scientific evidence.

Measuring psychoanalytic constructs

One of the major problems in the research literature on psychoanalysis is that clinical constructs need to be operationalized before they can be measured. This follows from a broad principle of science – one cannot study phenomena without first making them measurable. In psychology this usually means developing self-report measures.

Psychological research has great expertise in developing valid and reliable measures of mental activity. Observer-rated measures lead to problems because they use more time and require training. For example, one of the standard measures of attachment style, the Adult Attachment Interview (AAI; Main et al., 1985), is too complex for wide use in research.

Some researchers have attempted to square this circle, by developing self-report measures of key psychological constructs. For example, Sidney Blatt applied object relations theory and attachment theory to develop a way of measuring separate and distinct psychodynamic pathways to clinical depression (Blatt and Levy, 2003). Fonagy, Steele, Steele, and Target (1998) developed a *Reflective Functioning Questionnaire* (RFQ), which measures the ability of patients to observe themselves, related to the broader concept of mentalization (Bateman and Fonagy, 2004).

There have also been attempts to reconcile psychoanalytic theories of dreaming with scientific findings (Fonagy, 2003). This area reflects a great divide. Most of the researchers who discovered rapid-eye movement (a marker of dreaming) have never accepted Freud's approach (Hobson, 2015). It remains unclear whether the gap can be bridged. While the content of dreams is usually related to current life events, Freud's idea that they usually reflect wishes has not been supported by research.

One potentially productive line of investigation is the measurement of defense mechanisms. Originally considered as defenses against inner drives, these patterns are better conceptualized as coping mechanisms. A group at my department (Perry and Cooper, 1989; Bond, 2009), building on earlier work by the psychoanalyst George Vaillant (1994), has carried out extensive research on this subject. They showed that the defenses described by Freud can be measured with empirically validated self-report rating scales, and that patients move up a hierarchy to more healthy defenses when they improve. This is a good model for how complex and clinically derived concepts, even those that assume unconscious processes, can be operationalized for systematic research.

Approaches to measurement using projective tests runs into more serious difficulties. Thus, the Rorschach test remains controversial after nearly a century of work (Wood et al., 2003). The Thematic Apperception Test (TAT), using drawings instead of inkblots, also has major problems with validity and reliability (Lilienfeld et al., 2000). These instruments are rarely used today in research.

By and large, self-report measures are more valid measures of the mind than clinical judgment. One major objection of psychoanalysts to self-report, or even to observer-based ratings of psychological phenomena, is that they fail to capture the richness of mental activity. An example of the latter is the Diagnostic and Statistical Manual, 5th edition (American Psychiatric Association, 2013), which many analysts find naive and superficial. That view led to the creation of a Psychodynamic Diagnostic Manual (PDM-2, Lingiardi and McWiliams, 2017) to fill the gap. The problem is that ratings of psychodynamics by therapists may or may not be reliable, particularly when used by researchers or clinicians not involved with their development.

Is psychoanalytic treatment evidence-based?

This is a crucial issue in research on psychoanalysis. We now know that psychotherapy is usually effective for a wide range of problems (Smith et al., 1980; Lambert, 2013). All forms of therapy establish a therapeutic alliance, which describes how therapist and patients work actively on life problems; scales measuring the alliance are consistently correlated with a positive outcome (Lambert, 2013). Freud deserves credit for being among the first to understand that the therapeutic relationship is a powerful instrument for change, a principle that has been supported by many lines of research. On the other hand, there is more than one way of achieving the goal of establishing a strong alliance. This brings us to the domain of *process* research on psychotherapy, i.e., examining the mechanisms by which treatment helps patients.

We still lack precise knowledge about how therapy helps patients. There is also little evidence to support the view that any form of therapy, including psychoanalysis, has unique effects. Instead, a large body of research supports the conclusion that most forms of psychotherapy, whatever their theoretical basis, work in much the same way (Wampold, 2001). This result, one of the best supported empirical findings about psychotherapy, has sometimes been called a "dodo bird verdict" (echoing a scene from Lewis Carroll's Alice in Wonderland, where the dodo runs a race in which everyone wins and gets prizes).

The conclusion is that *common factors* – a positive relationship with a therapist, the promotion of hope, and the teaching of cognitive and interpersonal skills, are the crucial factors promoting psychological change, independent of theories adhered to by therapists. This is why researchers rarely find differences when therapies are compared head to head. And when you ask patients what happened in therapy, they talk about the treatment relationship, not the theory behind the method. This is what Strupp et al. (1969) observed in a study of how patients felt about the experience of receiving psychodynamic therapy.

Some of these common factors had been studied decades ago by the American psychologist Carl Rogers (1942), who described them as congruence: genuineness (openness and self-disclosure), acceptance (being seen with unconditional positive regard), and empathy (being listened to and understood). These "Rogerian" conditions are probably necessary but not sufficient for good psychotherapy. They do not mean that *any* method is as good as any other. What they do mean is that specific interventions, whether the interpretations of a psychoanalysts, or the cognitive schema favored by CBT therapists, are less powerful than an ability to form a strong alliance.

Consider, for example, the traditional emphasis in psychoanalytic therapy on interpreting transference. There has been some research on measuring this phenomenon, such as the Core Conflict Relationship Theme (CCRT; Luborsky and Barrett, 2006). Yet studies on the effectiveness of transference interpretations is at best mixed (Levy and Scala, 2012). Some data suggest that too much emphasis on the transference can be dangerous in less well-functioning patients (Piper et al., 1991). While it is useful to observe transference, there is no evidence that talking about it is uniquely effective. Another view would be to see transference as a way of monitoring the quality of the therapeutic relationship.

Moving from process to *outcome* research, all empirical studies of psychotherapy need to have a reliable way of establishing whether treatment is effective. One cannot simply assume that a therapy works because it fits a plausible theory, or because practitioners claim it to be effective, and write books about their methods. Nor is it sufficient to provide a few case reports to support broad conclusions. It is also not sufficient to rely entirely on pre-post comparisons without clinical trials. While effectiveness studies (measuring pre-post changes) can point in the right direction, one needs to follow up with efficacy research: conducting randomized clinical trials with a comparison to a control group.

The American Psychological Association uses this benchmark to determine whether any treatment can be considered an "empirically supported therapy" (EST). While this approach to validating therapy has had its critics (e.g., Wachtel, 2010), it is correctly considered to be a gold standard. Even better, since single studies are not always replicated, a meta-analysis of many studies is more convincing. Unfortunately, data has never been collected, and analyzed in this way, to assess the effects of classical psychoanalysis.

Modern medicine and psychiatry expect all forms of therapy to be based on high quality evidence. This usually means that treatment, whether a drug or a psychological intervention, should be supported by randomized clinical trials using comparison with a control group. Ideally, multiple studies can then be combined in metanalyses to see if they all point in the same direction. This is the method used by the Cochrane Reports, generally considered the gold standard for studies of medical and psychological treatments of all kinds.

Based on a very large body of systematic research, we can say that most people who embark on psychotherapy benefit from it (Lambert, 2013). But we need to bring the psychotherapy outcome literature into the theory and practice of psychoanalysis. Outcome research is a project that began as a response to a claim by the British psychologist Hans Eysenck (1952) that psychotherapy yielded no better outcomes than spontaneous recovery. His conclusion turned out to be wrong. And Eysenck later considered behavior therapy to be a panacea. Even so, he was a useful gadfly. Hundreds of systematic studies have now been conducted on the outcome of psychotherapy, using methods similar to those applied to clinical trials of drugs in medicine.

Eventually there was enough data to support a conclusion based on a large-scale metanalysis (Smith et al., 1980, p. 10): "Psychotherapy benefits people of all ages as reliably as school educates them, medicine cures them, or business turns a profit". That verdict still holds. Even if talking therapies are not always effective for treating psychological symptoms, they are as good in practice as practices that we consider routine.

There are now many thousands of research papers on psychotherapy, and they have been summarized in a standard handbook, now in its 6th edition (Lambert, 2013). Most research concerns other forms of talking therapy. Moreover, research supporting the effectiveness of *all* forms of psychotherapy is limited to brief treatment lasting for a few months. But not a single clinical trial using a control group has ever been conducted comparing a full course of psychoanalysis to no treatment, or to competing methods of treatment. All we have is pre-post (before and after) data. These *effectiveness* studies can be useful, but need to be bolstered by *efficacy* research (i.e., randomized clinical trials). No study has been able to answer the question of whether patients who undergo lengthy procedures get better, or if they do, simply improve with time, or might have benefited equally from brief treatment. Moreover, it is also difficult to conduct research in a large sample. For example, one of the few studies of outcome in long-term psychoanalytic therapy had only 30 subjects (Kachele et al., 2004).

The only study that has approached the problem with proper tools was derived from the Helsinki Psychotherapy Project (Jyra et al., 2017). This research examined improvements in overall health over five years, comparing results in 367 patients randomized to solution-focused therapy, short-term psychodynamic psychotherapy, and long-term psychodynamic psychotherapy. But the findings showed almost no differences between the groups. Similarly, when outcome of short-term and long-term psychodynamic therapy were compared after ten years, there were no differences (Knekt et al., 2016).

Crucially, research on the outcome of long-term psychoanalysis has relied almost entirely on effectiveness data, i.e., asking patients how they feel before and after the treatment. Such methods are unable to determine if clinical improvements are the result of therapy or intervening life events or maturation. The issue is partly practical: there are good efficacy studies (randomized clinical trials with control groups) of brief psychodynamic therapy lasting just a few months (Leichsenring et al., 2004), as well as a Cochrane report (Abbass et al., 2014) summarizing the literature and supporting the same conclusion.

It is problematic to assess the value of long-term therapy entirely on what patients say about it. This is a particular problem for evaluating therapies in which patients have made a large psychological and financial investment. For example, a survey of psychotherapies of various kinds, sponsored by the magazine *Consumer Reports*, found that most people who undergo treatment have mostly positive things to say about it, particularly when they spent more time in therapy (Seligman, 1995). While this was good to hear, it did not show that psychotherapy is better than no treatment, or that long-term therapy is best.

Again, we are faced with crucial unanswered questions. While research shows that brief psychotherapy is efficacious, does treatment have to last for years rather than months to be helpful? And is any one form of therapy that much better than any other?

In a research update on psychodynamic therapies, Fonagy (2015, p. 1137) remarked:

> The history of medicine is littered with interventions that did remarkable duty as therapies and yet, when subjected to RCT methodology, were shown either to have no benefit over alternative treatments or even to prevent the patient from benefiting, in terms of effect size or speed, from a superior intervention. Perhaps the most dramatic example is the RCT that ended 100 years of radical mastectomies for breast carcinoma only 30 years ago. The study showed that half a million women who had been subjected to disabling, mutilating operations, performed with the best of intentions on the basis of a fallacious theory about how carcinoma spreads, could have had equally good outcomes with lumpectomies.

Might these comments apply to classical psychoanalysis? In an earlier paper, Fonagy (2003, p. 77) acknowledged that "the evidence base for psychoanalytic therapy remains thin". A review chapter for which I was his co-author (Fonagy and Paris, 2008) concluded that much more research would be needed. In his most recent review, Fonagy (2015) was more optimistic, but almost all of the encouraging data he quoted was derived from studies of brief psychodynamic therapy.

At this point the only studies of the effectiveness of psychoanalysis have been pre-post. The Stockholm Outcome of Psychotherapy and Psychoanalysis Project (Sandell et al., 2000) examined the outcome of psychoanalysis or long-term psychodynamic therapy in 400 patients. But in spite of a large sample, its methods did not allow for firm conclusions. First and foremost, there was no control group. How can we know whether these patients would have improved with a briefer treatment, or with no treatment at all? Second, the data was entirely based on patient self-report.

The Stockholm study is not the only published research on the effectiveness of psychoanalysis. A few years ago, a meta-analysis of 14 studies was published, concluding (de Maat et al., 2013, p. 107):

> A limited number of mainly pre/post studies, presenting mostly completers analyses, provide empirical evidence for pre/post changes in psychoanalysis patients with complex mental disorders, but the lack of comparisons with control treatments is a serious limitation in interpreting the results.

Returning to the question of whether long-term psychoanalysis is preferable to brief therapy, or to therapies based on different theoretical frameworks, we also lack the data reach a conclusion. It is tempting but mistaken to generalize from evidence for the efficacy of short-term psychodynamic psychotherapy to support the practice of classical psychoanalysis. And given the evidence that different therapies produce very similar results, one cannot conclude that psychodynamic interventions are uniquely effective. As we have seen, patients do not necessarily agree with therapists that the interventions they value the most are crucial to recovery. Finally, therapies with different theoretical frameworks may be more similar than they appear. For example, helping patients understand how their past experiences affect the present is not unique to a psychodynamic method; CBT uses the construct of cognitive schemas to understand the impact of life histories.

Clearly, we need more research that specifically examines long-term treatment. The usual rationale for extended psychotherapy is for the treatment of complex but non-psychotic mental disorders, particularly personality disorders. Yet even these cases may respond more rapidly to therapy that clinicians expect.

Fonagy, in collaboration with the British analyst Anthony Bateman, has applied research methods to the treatment of complex problems such as personality disorders, developing a therapy they call "mentalization-based treatment" (MBT; Bateman and Fonagy, 2004). MBT is a combination of individual and group therapy that typically lasts for at least 18 months (which is long, but not nearly as long as classical psychoanalysis). Evidence from trials conducted both in day treatment and out-patient settings has supported the efficacy of their approach for personality disorders. Moreover, the MBT method, which teaches patients to identify their emotions as well as the feelings of other people, is an eclectic mixture of psychodynamic and cognitive behavioral interventions adapted for the treatment of severely ill patients.

MBT is a very creative idea, and its developers believe that increasing mentalization is a key mechanism in all kinds of psychotherapy. It parallels similar advances in cognitive therapy for personality disordered patients pioneered by the American psychologist Marsha Linehan (1993), whose method of dialectical behavior therapy (DBT) also uses individual and group therapy over at least a year. DBT has been supported by multiple clinical trials. But one cannot generalize from this research to conclude that long-term treatment is generally necessary. We do not know if patients would benefit just as much from a shorter and more focused course of treatment (Paris, 2017b).

The most serious attempt to demonstrate the value of longer treatment was carried out by the German psychoanalyst Falk Leichsenring, who published a series of meta-analyses of extended forms of psychoanalytic therapy (Leichsenring and Rabung, 2008, 2011). The first of these papers attracted particular attention because it was published in the *Journal of the American Medical Association* (*JAMA*). Leichensring and his colleagues claimed that research supports long-term treatment for complex mental disorders, such as personality disorders.

However, these conclusions were not convincing, as noted by several critics (Bhar et al., 2010; Anestis et al., 2011). The problems arise from the limitations of their meta-analysis, combining data from heterogeneous clinical presentations in small samples, and with findings that are limited by small effect sizes. Essentially, these meta-analyses combine data from many weak studies, which does not make for strong conclusions. While some researchers (Shedler, 2010) have argued that the Leichsenring studies support the efficacy of longer periods of psychodynamic therapy for complex disorders, the evidence is not strong.

To show that long-term therapies are necessary would require another kind of research design, in which patients are randomly assigned therapy of shorter and longer duration. This kind of research is very rare. One of my Canadian colleagues, Shelley McMain, is currently carrying out a study of this kind on dialectical behavior therapy. Fonagy et al. (2015) reported that in patients with treatment-resistant depression, a longer course (18 months) produced a better result (with one-third of the cohort going into remission) than in the group randomized to brief therapy. This study does suggest that some patients do need longer treatment, although its findings cannot be generalized to most of the patients that clinicians see.

In a comprehensive review of the literature, Barber et al. (2013) noted that there is strong evidence from several metanalyses for the efficacy of short-term dynamic therapy in depression, anxiety, and personality disorders. However, the authors failed to find convincing evidence supporting the use of open-ended long-term therapy. While a research group supported by the International Psychoanalytic Association (Leuzinger-Bohleben and Kachele, 2016) came to more positive conclusions, the data base they used consisted entirely of pre-post-comparisons. One would like to see this question addressed by the Cochrane Collaboration, which requires efficacy based on clinical trials, and on meta-analyses of these trials. But in the absence of such evidence, Cochrane has never published guidelines on the clinical use of psychoanalysis.

Admittedly, it is difficult to conduct a clinical trial of any treatment that lasts for years. (And who would be in the control group?) For all these reasons, a convincing study of outcome might be impossibly expensive, and unlikely to be funded. Nonetheless, given that time-limited psychoanalytic therapy already has a strong evidence base, it should be a better alternative for most patients than long-term, open-ended treatment.

Some of the same problems can be described in the literature on cognitive behavioral therapy. Like psychoanalysis, CBT was originally developed as a brief therapy, but became longer with time. Its current dominance is based on the very large number of studies supporting it. Almost all these studies are short-term. And when it comes to brief therapy, the psychodynamic approach is as efficacious as CBT (Goodyer et al., 2017). As

Shedler (2010) correctly points out, the evidence base for psychoanalytic therapy is as good as that for CBT; but it took a very long time for research to get started.

Another problem with psychotherapies is that therapists in practice, whatever their orientation, eventually run into the problem of "interminability" (Freud, 1937). I have seen CBT therapists, just like psychoanalysts, continue seeing patients for years. If patients do not meet their goals, they are kept on in the hope that they eventually will. In Chapter 5, I will discuss how to make the goals of therapy more realistic.

The movement to integrate psychotherapy

As psychoanalysis has evolved, its theories have been modified, and will no doubt be further modified. For both theoretical and empirical reasons, the most important revision has been attachment theory (see Chapter 3). Practice has also evolved, with classical methods replaced by therapies of lower frequency and shorter duration. More patients now receive time-limited treatment, and when therapy is open-ended, patients are usually seen once a week. In a recent review of research on psychodynamic therapy, Barber et al. (2013) commented that: "psychodynamic therapy . . . did not disappear but sprouted many variations and new offspring. Today those offspring have forgotten everything about their origins".

In spite of many changes, the ideas of Sigmund Freud left an important legacy to clinical psychology and psychiatry (Lacewing, 2013). Psychoanalysis taught a generation of therapists how to understand life histories, and how to listen attentively to what patients say about their lives. By considering the person, and not just the symptom, it introduced humanism into mental health practice. Moreover, many of its ideas are integral parts of competing forms of therapy (Shedler, 2010).

In the current context of mental health treatment, psychotherapies of all kinds have become increasingly marginal to the practice of psychiatry. Surveys show that psychiatrists offer less psychotherapy and have been concentrating on pharmacological methods (Olfson et al., 2002). Many clinicians have fallen back on their medical training to embrace neuroscience – and neuroscience alone – as the basis of their practice. Today patients who are treated by psychiatrists tend to receive diagnoses that are based on symptom checklists, and may be prescribed interventions consisting of aggressive forms of pharmacology (Paris, 2017a). These procedures may work for severe forms of mental illness, but not for the problems for which most people seek help. As a result, patients are not getting the care and understanding they need.

Clinical psychology, a discipline that now dominates the practice of psychotherapy, presents a different set of problems. Hundreds of different methods of therapy have been described, with brand names that are marketed using catchy acronyms. (This trend has ironically been called "acronym-based treatment".) Yet there is no evidence that trendy treatments, such as Acceptance and Commitment Therapy (ACT, Hayes et al., 2012), or Eye Movement Desensitization and Reprocessing (EMDR, Bradley et al., 2005), offer better results than standard methods. Another irony is that even as they proclaim their separateness, the latest brands of therapy all make use of principles derived from psychoanalysis.

As we have seen, research shows that there are few differences in efficacy between specific psychotherapy methods, suggesting that *common factors* are more important than specific techniques in predicting positive outcomes. For example, there is no difference in outcome between short-term dynamic therapy and a brief course of CBT, either in adults (Goldstone, 2016; Gibbons et al., 2016), or in adolescents (Goodyer et al., 2017). Kagan (2017, p. 60) makes the following observation:

> Psychoanalysts require patients to lie on a couch and free-associate. This form of therapy was {considered} successful for about 50 years. After the rituals had lost their novelty, both clients and analysts lost some faith in the curative power of the procedure. The rituals of psychoanalytic therapy are novel to contemporary Chinese, and wealthy Chinese are seeking this form of therapy. Cognitive behavioral therapy (CBT) has been a popular treatment for depression for about the same length of time. Recent evaluations, however, reveal that it is no more or less effective than any form of dynamic psychotherapy with an experienced therapist.

How then does psychotherapy work? Basically, by establishing a therapeutic alliance so that patients get on the same page of their therapist, by establishing trust so that patients can discuss personal issues with comfort, and by focusing on current interpersonal problems while making suggestions of how relationships can be improved. These are some of the common factors in all effective therapies (Wampold, 2001). But there is no research evidence that specific interventions, whether transference interpretations or elucidation of cognitive schemas, are in any way as central to the outcome of treatment.

These research findings are the basis of a movement for *psychotherapy integration* (Norcross and Goldfried, 2005). The implication is that therapists should use the best ideas from all methods of therapy, and combine them in packages that yield the best results. These principles have been developed by the Society for the Exploration of Psychotherapy Integration (SEPI), which also sponsors a *Journal of Psychotherapy Integration*.

This approach could well be useful for integrating psychodynamic treatments with other forms of therapy. As Bateman (2002, p. 11) comments:

> Unable to consider new findings and fresh ideas, particularly from cognitive theory and cognitive-behaviour therapy, psychoanalysis is in danger not only of becoming intellectually isolated but also of becoming a body of knowledge uninfluenced by and unable to influence other disciplines. In the end this weakens its own development, impoverishes that of others and is likely to discourage the cross-fertilization that would benefit both parent and offspring.

Applying integration to the therapy of personality disorders

The treatment of borderline personality disorder (BPD), my own area of specialization, is a good example of integration in psychotherapy. This complex disorder was first described by a psychoanalyst (Stern, 1938). Once considered relatively untreatable, BPD has now attracted a set of methods for management, each of which has earned support from clinical trials. The best known is dialectical behavior therapy (DBT), a method derived from CBT, focusing on developing skills in emotion regulation (Linehan, 1993). Actually, DBT has several points in common with psychodynamic therapy, in that it promotes self-observation on the part of the patient, aims to ensure that the therapist is empathic (a process termed "validation"), and encourages patients to move beyond their past experiences (a process termed "radical acceptance").

Another method of treating BPD, Transference-Focused Psychotherapy (TFP), is directly derived from psychoanalytic methods. Based on ideas developed by Otto Kernberg, it uses transference in the therapy sessions to illustrate and modify problematic interpersonal patterns; it has been also been supported by clinical trials (Yeomans et al., 2015).

Mentalization-based treatment (MBT, Bateman and Fonagy, 2004) can best be described as using psychoanalytic concepts associated with the theory of mind, as well as cognitive concepts (using mentalization to improve emotional control and to develop better interpersonal skills). MBT is a good example of psychotherapy integration. It was developed by two psychoanalysts but applies cognitive theory, using a combination of group and individual therapy. Its emphasis on accurate observation of emotions in self and others (mentalization) is similar both to psychodynamic ideas such as the observing ego and to DBT's use of techniques to promote "mindfulness". It has been shown to be superior to treatment in a control group using general approaches to practice (Bateman and Fonagy, 2004).

Other options for the treatment of BPD include Schema Focused Therapy, a combination of psychodynamic and cognitive therapy (Arntz, 2012), and Good Psychiatric Management (GPM), an eclectic therapy developed by a psychoanalyst, John Gunderson (Gunderson and Links, 2014). There is also a short-term group therapy designed for regions where psychotherapists are rare (Systems Training for Emotional Predictability and Problem Solving; Black and Blum, 2017). All these methods, while derived from different traditions, have points of commonality with psychoanalysis.

Our own programs for BPD, described in a recent book (Paris, 2017b), also make use of ideas from many sources, combining ideas from DBT, MBT, and GPM. We definitely make use of psychodynamic concepts, but unlike previous treatments for this population, therapy is time-limited and goal directed.

Conclusion

The original version of psychoanalysis must now be considered more historical than current. Westen (1998) made a strong argument that given the revisions that have emerged in the model, given the empirical support for some of its principles, and given that brief courses of psychodynamic therapy are effective, clinical psychology should remain informed by psychodynamic principles. But none of these ideas will be widely accepted unless they can be rooted in systematic research. Several observers (Chiesa, 2010; Kernberg, 2015) have described the unreasonable resistance to research among senior analysts, and have argued for the building of a bridge between empirical and clinical domains.

Psychoanalysis cannot remain isolated. It needs to rejoin the mainstream of scientific research (Bornstein, 2005). It must embrace the malleability of science, remaining open to change over time as new data come in that can change paradigms. Chapter 4 will suggest ways in which research is relevant to developing a different, more integrated kind of clinical practice.

References

Abbass, A.A., Kisely, S.R., Town, J.M., Leichsenring, F., Driessen, E., De Maat, S., Gerber, A., Dekker, J., Rabung, S., Rusalovska, S., Crowe, E.: Short-term psychodynamic psychotherapies for common mental disorders. *Cochrane Database of Systematic Reviews* 2014, (7). Art. No.: CD004687.

American Psychiatric Association: *Diagnostic and Statistical Manual of Mental Disorders*, 5th edition. Washington, DC, American Psychiatric Publishing, 2013.

Anestis, M.D., Anestis, J., Lilienfeld, S.O.: When it comes to evaluating psychodynamic therapy, the devil is in the details. *American Psychologist* 2011, 66: 149–151.

Arntz, A.: A systematic review of schema therapy for BPD. In J.M. Farrell, I.A. Shaw, eds.: *Group Schema Therapy for Borderline Personality Disorder*. New York, Wiley, 2012, pp. 286–294.

Barber, J.P., Muran, J.C., McCarthy, K.S., Keefe, J.R.: Research on dynamic therapies. In M.J. Lambert, ed.: *Bergin and Garfield's Handbook of Psychotherapy and Behavior Change*. New York, Wiley, 2013, pp. 443–494.

Bargh, J.: *Before You Know It: The Unconscious Reasons Why We Do What We Do*. New York, Simon and Schuster, 2017.

Bateman, A.: Integration from an analytic perspective. In J. Holmes, A. Bateman, eds.: *Integration in Psychotherapy: Models and Methods*. Oxford, Oxford University Press, 2002.

Bateman, A., Fonagy, P.: *Psychotherapy for Borderline Personality Disorder: Mentalization Based Treatment*. Oxford, Oxford University Press, 2004.

Belsky, J., Pluess, M.: Beyond diathesis stress: Differential susceptibility to environmental Influences. *Psychological Bulletin* 2009, 135: 885–908.

Bhar, S.S., Thombs, B.D., Pignotti, M., Bassel, M., Jewett, L., Coyne, J., Beck, A.T.: Is longer-term psychodynamic psychotherapy more effective than shorter-term therapies? Review and critique of the evidence.*Psychotherapy and Psychosomatics*2010, 79: 208–216.

Black, D.W., Blum, N., eds.: *Systems Training for Emotional Predictability and Problem Solving for Borderline Personality Disorder: Implementing STEPPS Around the Globe*. New York, Oxford University Press, 2017.

Blatt, S., Levy, K.: Psychoanalysis, personality development, and psychopathology. *Psychoanalytic Inquiry* 2003, 23: 102–150.

Bond, M.: Empirical studies of defense style: Relationships with psychopathology and change. *Harvard Review of Psychiatry* 2009, 12: 263–278.

Bornstein, R.F.: Reconnecting psychoanalysis to mainstream psychology: Challenges and opportunities. *Psychoanalytic Psychology* 2005, 22: 323–340.

Bornstein, R.F., Masling, J.R.: *Empirical Perspectives on the Psychoanalytic Unconscious*. Washington, DC, American Psychological Association, 1998.

Bower, G.H.: Awareness, the unconscious, and repression. In J. Singer, ed.: *Repression and Dissociation: Implications for Personality Theory, Psychopathology, and Health*. Chicago, University of Chicago Press, 1990, pp. 209–231.

Bradley, R., Greene, J., Russ, E., Dutra, L., Westen, D.: A multidimensional meta-analysis of psychotherapy for PTSD. *American Journal of Psychiatry* 2005, 162: 214–227.

Chiesa, M.: Research and psychoanalysis: Still time to bridge the great divide? *Psychoanalytic Psychology* 2010, 27: 99–114.

Damasio, A.: *Descartes' Error: Emotion, Reason, and the Human Brain*. New York, Revised Penguin Edition, 2005.

Dehaene, J.P.: *Consciousness and the Brain*. New York, Penguin, 2014.

de Maat, S., Jonge, F., de Kraker, T., Leichsenring, F., Abbass, A., Luyten, P., Barber, J.P., Dekker, J.: The current state of the empirical evidence for psychoanalysis: A meta-analytic approach. *Harvard Review of Psychiatry* 2013, 21: 107–137.

Eagle, M.: *From Classical to Contemporary Psychoanalysis: A Critique and Integration*. New York, Routledge, 2011.

Eagle, M.: Attachment theory and research and clinical work. *Psychoanalytic Inquiry* 2017, 37: 284–297.

Ellenberger, H.: *The Discovery of the Unconscious*. New York, Basic Books, 1970.

Ellis, B.J., Boyce, W.T., Belsky, J, Bakermans-Kranenburg, M.J., va Ijzjendoorn, M.H.: Differential susceptibility to the environment: An evolutionary–neurodevelopmental theory. *Development and Psychopathology* 2011, 23: 7–28

Erikson, E.: *Childhood and Society*. New York, Norton, 1950.

Eysenck, H.: The effects of psychotherapy: An evaluation. *Journal of Consulting Psychology* 1952, 16: 319–324.

Fisher, S., Greenberg, R.P.: *Freud Scientifically Reappraised*. New York, Wiley, 1996.

Fonagy, P.: Genetics, developmental psychopathology, and psychoanalytic theory: The case for ending our (not so) splendid isolation. *Psychoanalytic Inquiry* 2003, 23: 239–247.

Fonagy, P.: The effectiveness of psychodynamic psychotherapies: An update. *World Psychiatry* 2015, 14: 1137–1150.

Fonagy, P.: Kachele, H., Leuzinger-Bohleber, M., Taylor, P.: *The Significance of Dreams: Bridging Clinical and Extraclinical Research in Psychoanalysis*. London, Karnac Books, 2012.

Fonagy, P., Paris, J.: Psychological treatments. In P. Tyrer, K. Silk, eds.: *Cambridge Handbook of Evidence-Based Psychiatric Treatment*. Cambridge, Cambridge University Press, 2008, pp. 98–115.

Fonagy, P., Rost, F., Carlyle, J.A., McPHersonm, S., Thomas, R., Pasco-Fearon, R.M., Goldberg, D., Taylor, D.: Pragmatic randomized controlled trial of long-term psychoanalytic psychotherapy for treatment-resistant depression: The Tavistock Adult Depression Study (TADS). *World Psychiatry* 2015, 14: 312–321.

Fonagy, P., Steele, M., Steele, H., Target, M.: *Reflexive-Function Manual: Version 5.0 for Application to the Adult Attachment Interview*. Unpublished manual, University College, London, 1998.

Freud, S.: Analysis terminable and Interminable. *International Journal of Psychoanalysis* 1937, 18: 373–385.

Gibbons, M.B.C., Gallop, R., Thompson, D.: Comparative effectiveness of cognitive therapy and dynamic psychotherapy for major depressive disorder in a community mental health setting: A randomized clinical non-inferiority trial. *JAMA Psychiatry* 2016, 73: 904–912.

Goldstone, D.: Cognitive-behavioural therapy versus psychodynamic psychotherapy for the treatment of depression: A critical review of evidence and current issues. *South African Journal of Psychology* 2016, 47: 1–22.

Goodyer, I., Reynolds, S., Barrett, B., Byford, A., Fonagy, P.: Cognitive behavioral therapy and short-term psychoanalytic psychotherapy versus a brief psychosocial intervention in adolescents with unipolar major depressive disorder. *Lancet Psychiatry* 2017, 4: 109–119.

Gunderson, J.G., Links, P.R.: *Handbook of Good Psychiatric Management for Borderline Personality Disorder*. Washington, DC, American Psychiatric Publishing, 2014.

Hayes, S.C., Strosahl, K.D., Wilson, K.G.: *Acceptance and Commitment Therapy: The Process and Practice of Mindful Change*, 2nd edition. New York, Guilford Press, 2012.

Hobson, J.A.: *Psychodynamic Neurology: Dreams, Consciousness, and Virtual Reality*. New York, Taylor & Francis, 2015.

Hume, D.: *A Treatise of Human Nature*. London, Longmans, Green & Co, 1739/1882.

Jang, K.L.: *The Behavior Genetics of Psychopathology*. New York, Taylor & Francis, 2008.

Jyra, K., Knekt, P., LIndfors, O.: The impact of psychotherapy treatments of different length and type on health behaviour during a five-year follow-up. *Psychotherapy Research* 2017, 4: 397–409.

Kachele, H., Renlund, C., Richardson, P.: *Research on Psychoanalytic Psychotherapy with Adults*. London, Karnak, 2004.

Kagan, J.: *Three Seductive Ideas*. Cambridge, MA, Harvard University Press, 1998.

Kagan, J.: *An Argument for Mind*. New Haven, Yale University Press, 2006.

Kagan, J.: *Five Constraints on Predicting Behavior*. Cambridge, MA, MIT Press, 2017.

Kahnemann, D.: *Thinking Fast and Slow*. New York, Palgrave MacMillan, 2011.

Kernberg, O.F.: Resistances and progress in developing a research framework in psychoanalytic institutes. *Psychoanalytic Inquiry* 2015, 35, suppl 1: 98–114.

Kihlstrom, J.F.: The cognitive unconscious. *Science* 1987, 237: 1445–1452.

Kihlstrom, J.F.: Dynamic versus cognitive unconscious. In S.O. LIlienfeld, R.L. Cautin, eds.: *The Encyclopedia of Clinical Psychology*. New York, Wiley-Blackwell, 2015, pp. 1–8.

Knekt, P., Virtala, E., Harkanen, T., Vaarama, M.: The outcome of short- and long-term psychotherapy 10 years after start of treatment. *Psychological Medicine* 2016, 46: 1175–1188.

Lacewing, M.: Could psychoanalysis be a science? In K.W.M. Fulford, M. Davies, R. Gipps, G. Graham, J.Z. Sadler, G. Stanghellini, T. Thornton, eds.: *The Oxford Handbook of Philosophy and Psychiatry*. New York, Oxford University Press, 2013, pp. 1103–1127.

Lambert, M.J.: *Bergin and Garfield's Handbook of Psychotherapy and Behavior Change*. New York, Wiley, 2013.

Lane, R.D., Ryan, L., Nadel, L., Greenberg, L.: Memory reconsolidation, emotional arousal, and the process of change in psychotherapy: New insights from brain science. *Behavioral and Brain Sciences* 2015, 38: 1–80.

Leichsenring, F., Rabung, S.: Effectiveness of long-term psychodynamic psychotherapy: A meta-analysis. *JAMA* 2008, 300: 1551–1565.

Leichsenring, F., Rabung, S.: Long-term psychodynamic psychotherapy in complex mental disorders: Update of a meta-analysis. *British Journal of Psychiatry* 2011, 199: 15–22.

Leichsenring, F., Rabung, S., Leibing, E.: The efficacy of short-term psychodynamic psychotherapy in specific psychiatric disorders: A meta-analysis. *Archives of General Psychiatry* 2004, 61: 1208–1216.

Leuzinger-Bohleben, M., Kachele, H., eds.: *An Open Door Review of Outcome and Process Studies in Psychoanalysis*, 3rd edition. London, International Psychoanalytic Association, 2016.

Levy, K.N., Scala, J.W.: Transference, transference interpretations, and transference-focused psychotherapies. *Psychotherapy* 2012, 49: 391–403.

Lilienfeld, S.O., Wood, J.M., Garb, H.N.: The scientific status of projective techniques. *Psychological Science in the Public Interest* 2000, 1: 27–66.

Linehan, M.M.: *Cognitive-Behavioral Treatment of Borderline Personality Disorder*. New York, Guilford Press, 1993.

Lingiardi, V., McWiliams, N.: *Psychodynamic Diagnostic Manual*, 2nd edition. New York, Guilford Press, 2017.

Loftus, E.F., Ketcham, K.: *The Myth of Repressed Memory*. New York, St. Martin's Press, 1994.

Luborsky, L., Barrett, M.: The history and empirical status of key psychoanalytic concepts. *Annual Review of Clinical Psychology* 2006, 2: 1–19.

Main, M., Kaplan, N., Cassidy, J.: Security in infancy, childhood, and adulthood: A move to the level of representation. *Monographs of the Society for Research in Child Development* 1985, 50: 66–104.

Norcross, J.C., Goldfried, M.R.: *Handbook of Psychotherapy Integration*. New York, Oxford University Press, 2005.

Olfson, M., Marcus, S.M., Druss, B., Pincus, H.A.: National trends in the use of outpatient psychotherapy. *American Journal of Psychiatry* 2002, 159: 1914–1920.

Paris, J.: *Myths of Childhood*. Philadelphia, Brunner/Mazel, 2000.

Paris, J.: *Psychotherapy in an Age of Neuroscience*. New York, Oxford University Press, 2017a.

Paris, J.: *Stepped Care for Borderline Personality Disorder: Making Treatment Brief, Effective, and Accessible*. New York, Academic Press/Elsevier, 2017b.

Perry, J.C., Cooper, S.H.: An empirical study of defense mechanisms. *Archives of General Psychiatry* 1989, 46: 444–452.

Piper, W.E., Azim, H.F., Joyce, A.S., McCallum, M.: Transference interpretations, therapeutic alliance, and outcome in short-term individual psychotherapy. *Archives of General Psychiatry* 1991, 48: 946–953.

Plomin, R., DeFries, J.C., Knopik, V.S., Neiderhiser, J.M.: *Behavioral Genetics*, 6th edition. London, UK, Worth, 2012.

Rogers, C.: *Counseling and Psychotherapy: Newer Concepts in Practice*. New York, Houghton Mifflin, 1942.

Rutter, M.J.: Resilience as a dynamic concept. *Development and Psychopathology* 2012a, 24: 335–334.

Rutter, M.J.: Gene-environment interdependence. *European Journal of Developmental Psychology* 2012b, 9: 391–412.

Rutter, M.J., Rutter, M.J.: *Developing Minds: Challenge and Continuity across the Life Span*. New York, Basic Books, 1993.

Sandell, R., Bloomberg, J., Lazar, A., Carlson, J., Broberg, J.: Varieties of long-term outcome among patients in psychoanalysis and long-term psychotherapy: A review of findings in the Stockholm Outcome of Psychoanalysis and Psychotherapy Project (STOPP). *International Journal of Psychoanalysis* 2000, 81: 921–942.

Schacter, D.L.: *Searching for Memory: The Brain, the Mind, and the Past.* New York, Basic Books, 1995.

Schacter, D.L.: *Searching for Memory: The Brain, the Mind, and the Past.* New York, Basic Books, 2008.

Seligman, M.: The effectiveness of psychotherapy: The consumer reports study. *American Psychologist* 1995, 50: 965–974.

Shedler, J.: The efficacy of psychodynamic psychotherapy. *American Psychologist* 2010, 65: 98–109.

Smith, M.L., Glass, G.V., Miller, T.: *The Benefits of Psychotherapy.* Baltimore, Johns Hopkins Press, 1980.

Stern, A.: Psychoanalytic investigation of and therapy in the borderline group of neuroses. *Psychoanalytic Quarterly* 1938, 7: 467–489.

Strupp, H.H., Fox, R.E., Lessler, K.: *Patients View Their Psychotherapy.* Baltimore, Johns Hopkins Press, 1969.

Thaler, R.: *Misbehaving: The Story of Behavioral Economics.* New York, Norton, 2015.

Wachtel, P.: Beyond "ESTs": Problematic assumptions in the pursuit of evidence-based practice. *Psychoanalytic Psychology* 2010, 27: 151–172.

Wampold, B.E.: *The Great Psychotherapy Debate: Models, Methods, and Findings.* Mahwah, NJ, Erlbaum Associates, 2001.

Westen, D.: The scientific legacy of Sigmund Freud: Towards a psychodynamically informed psychological science. *Psychological Bulletin* 1998, 124: 128–136.

Wood, J.M., Nezworski, M.T., Lillienfeld, S.O., Garb, H.: *What's Wrong with the Rorschach.* San Francisco, Jossey-Bass, 2003.

Woodhouse, S., Miah, A., Rutter, M.: A new look at the supposed risks of early institutional rearing. *Psychological Medicine* 2017, 42: 1–10.

Yeomans, F.E., Clarkin, J.F., Kernberg, O.F.: *Transference-Focused Psychotherapy for Borderline Personality Disorder: A Clinical Guide.* Washington, DC, American Psychiatric Publishing, 2015.

Chapter 3

Changing the paradigm

Revisions of psychoanalytic theory

Psychoanalysis, like any other scientific theory, has undergone revision over time. One would not judge physics or biology by ideas that were current a century ago. Even if Freud's original ideas have not gained consistent support from empirical research, newer models of psychoanalysis could be more compatible with empirical findings.

Freud's original theory had many problems. Crucially, his hypothesis that childhood sexuality lies at the core of personality and psychopathology has not been backed up by research, nor has his focus on drives and intrapsychic conflict gained empirical support (Fisher and Greenberg, 1996). Over the years, many revisions have been proposed to expand the framework of analytic theory. Most of them have modified the theory to downplay sexuality and drives, underlining the crucial role of interpersonal relations, both during development, and in adult life (Eagle, 2014).

Some of these revisions go back many decades. In the USA, a group of "neo-Freudians", including Karen Horney (1940), Erich Fromm (1940), and Harry Stack Sullivan (1953), eliminated drive theory and emphasized how interpersonal relationships, as well as social forces, shape symptoms. Later, a similar set of ideas, called "ego psychology" (Blanck and Blanck, 1994), was notable for downplaying traumas in the past, focusing on coping in the present.

These trends were combined in what has been called *relational psychoanalysis* (Greenberg and Mitchell, 1983). Influenced by the Scottish analyst Ronald Fairbairn (1952), Stephen Mitchell proposed an American version of an approach developed in the UK. Mitchell, influential in clinical psychology as a teacher, was also involved with the William Alanson White Institute, a group founded by a group of neo-Freudians who stood outside the mainstream of psychoanalysis. Mitchell had the specific goal of moving the perspective of psychoanalysis from the intrapsychic to the interpersonal. For this reason, the relational movement does a better rob of reflecting what therapy is about, and has been influential among clinicians (Mills, 2005, 2012). However, neither its theory nor its method have ever been assessed in formal research.

Another construct promoting the replacement of drive theory by a more interpersonal model was *self-psychology*. This was the brain-child of the Austrian-American analyst Heinz Kohut (1970). In this theory, adult psychological problems, particularly pathological narcissism, were attributed largely to a failure of "mirroring", i.e., a mother's approving interest in a child's feelings. The implication for practice involved offering accurate empathy to patients who deal with their inner emptiness by embracing grandiosity. For a time, self-psychology was the "latest thing" in psychoanalysis. In the 1970s, several colleagues in my department would fly to Chicago once every two weeks to obtain direct supervision from Kohut. Not for the first or last time, a revised version of psychoanalysis depended on following a charismatic clinician.

Kohut, who had been a leader in American psychoanalysis, tried to soft-pedal his differences from classical theory, suggesting that nothing need be removed, only that new perspectives can be added (Kohut, 1970). But some of Kohut's followers, e.g., Arnold Goldberg (1990), were openly critical of classical psychoanalysis, and considered self-psychology to be its replacement. A senior analyst in Montreal, one of the commuters to Chicago, told me that Kohut was to Freud what Einstein had been to Newton, by replacing an older paradigm with a newer one. (I suggested that a better analogy might be a shift from Plato to Aristotle.). However, Kohut's group had no tradition of empiricism, and his theories never stimulated a research program to determine whether its treatment method is superior. Decades later, researchers began to study narcissism more systematically, but their conclusions provided only partial support to the self-psychology model (Campbell and Miller, 2011).

In some ways, self-psychology bore a similarity to the ideas of the American psychologist Carl Rogers (1942), who had also worked in Chicago, and who developed a non-psychoanalytic method called *client-centered psychotherapy*. But in contrast to Kohut, Rogers's group conducted empirical research, showing that accurate empathy predicts a positive outcome in psychotherapy (Truax and Carkhuff, 1967).

The concept of mirroring also has a resemblance to the ideas of a cognitive behavioral therapist, Marsha Linehan (1993), who developed *dialectical behavior therapy* (DBT). While her model was not psychodynamic, Linehan hypothesized that *invalidation* of emotions (by families) is a major risk factor for the development of borderline personality disorder. Her view of this disorder was that when feelings are invalidated, children who are emotionally dysregulated can develop serious psychopathology. Much like Kohut, Linehan's therapy places a central emphasis on the ability of parents to understand feelings in their children. Linehan's ideas have stimulated a good deal of research, including her own studies showing that DBT is an efficacious treatment for chronically suicidal patients with borderline personality disorder. (Although Linehan might not admit it, she added a psychodynamic element to the narrower perspective of CBT.)

In the UK, other streams of thought deviated from classical analysis. One, developed by the Hungarian psychoanalyst Melanie Klein (Grosskurth, 1984), can be dismissed on the grounds that from the point of view of empirical science, it moved in the wrong direction. Klein proposed that problems in adulthood were largely related to intrapsychic conflicts in infancy. But since she exclusively depended on clinical methods, no researchable hypotheses emerged that could have tested her theory. Moreover, while many of Klein's ideas were based on what she called "infant observation", they actually consisted only of speculations about what infants *might* be thinking.

A more fertile line of theory was developed by the British school of object relations, which paralleled relational psychoanalysis. These ideas are associated with the work of Ronald Fairbairn (1952), Harry Guntrip (1969), and Donald Winnicott (1958). These analysts downplayed the role of sexuality and aggression, and emphasized interpersonal issues, which they saw as related to problems in the relation of a child to its mother. Therapists still talk of Winnicott's idea that what children need most is "good enough mothering". The attachment model arose out of that perspective, but eventually evolved into something rather different.

Thus most of the revisions of psychoanalysis moved in the direction of making theory and practice more relational and interpersonal. Given that problems with other people are the main reason why patients seek therapy, this shift is both logical and clinically relevant.

Yet there is still a big problem. Neither neo-Freudian models, nor ego psychology, nor relational psychoanalysis, nor self-psychology, have ever conducted empirical investigations of their theories, or of the process and outcome of the treatment approaches derived from these ideas. In the present climate of clinical care, where evidence-based methods are take precedence over speculation, the absence of supporting data means that these ideas remain out of the academic mainstream. This may explain why, after a period of initial enthusiasm, many of these alternative paradigms lost traction.

Attachment theory

Attachment theory, the brain-child of the British psychoanalyst John Bowlby (1969), is clearly the most important revision of psychoanalysis. Today, the theory has come to dominate the thinking of many analysts and psychodynamically oriented therapists (Holmes, 2014).

For one thing, the attachment model corresponds more closely to common sense, making few assumptions about intrapsychic processes, and linking real life events to measurable consequences. An even more important reason for its success is that attachment theory is the one version of psychoanalysis that has been made testable, and that has earned strong empirical support (Cassidy and Shaver, 2015).

Eagle (2014) has summarized some of the key findings from research on the attachment model. First, children have a need to stay close to caregivers. Second, secure attachments promote emotional regulation. Third, psychopathology is often associated with early separation, neglect, or maltreatment. Fourth, failure of secure attachment is associated with deficits in cognitive and social functioning. Fifth, at least to some extent, problems in attachment during childhood are associated with problems in adulthood.

Attachment theory has been considered by some to be at least partly distinct from psychoanalysis (Eagle, 2014). For example, it considers attachment between infants and their mothers to be a product of biological evolution, and not dependent (as Freud thought) on feeding. This explains why, in a famous experiment, monkeys separated from their mothers prefer to cling to a soft piece of cloth to a metal wire, even if the "wire mother" is the one that feeds them (Harlow, 1958). The attachment model also explains why children who are rejected by a parent will try even harder to gain love (something we see every day in the clinic when intimate relationships fail). Thus, the model rejects drive theories, and bases its conclusions on empirical evidence, evolutionary theory, and systems theory. Of clinical significance, the model puts more emphasis on real life experience than on fantasy.

Early on, Bowlby teamed up with the Canadian-American psychologist Mary Ainsworth (Ainsworth et al., 1978), who developed a way of testing hypotheses about attachment using "the strange situation", in which children were observed dealing with the absence and return of their mother. Crucially, these responses could be observed and converted into reliable scores.

Depending on their behavior in the strange situation, attachment patterns in children can be described as using four "styles": secure (the most common pattern), anxious-ambivalent, anxious-avoidant, or disorganized-disoriented. Later, the model was applied to adults, using Mary Main's Adult Attachment Interview (Main et al., 2008), an interview-based measure that can score attachment patterns in adult life.

Bowlby (1969, 1973, 1980) published three volumes on his theory (focusing, respectively on attachment, separation, and loss). In the 1970s, I read these books as they came out, and was greatly inspired by these ideas. Here was a man who took science seriously, and here was a psychoanalyst who actually quoted research – and did so on every page. Moreover, Bowlby made a serious attempt to make his theory compatible with evolutionary psychology (emphasizing the survival value of bonding to the mother), and with general systems theory (allowing for multiple effects that produce multiple outcomes).

Not every psychoanalyst shared my enthusiasm. Anna Freud, loyal to her father, never accepted Bowlby's model (Edgcumbe, 2001). Decades later, Fonagy and Campbell (2015) could still write about the "bad blood" between psychoanalysis and attachment theory. But unlike classical analysis, which has shown insufficient interest in scientific investigation, attachment theory stimulated many research studies (over 12,000 listed on PsycInfo). *The Handbook of Attachment*, now in its third edition (Cassidy and Shaver, 2015), is a large volume that summarizes this large body of investigation.

As a result of its strong base in research, the attachment model has been incorporated into developmental psychology. It is also in concord with revisions to classical psychoanalysis, as well as similar concepts derived from CBT. Within psychoanalysis, it has been suggested by attachment researchers that *mentalization*, the ability to identify emotions in self or others, is a key issue in development and in psychotherapy (Fonagy and

Allison, 2014). In CBT, the related concept of *cognitive schemas* is a useful way of thinking about how early experiences affect adult behavior (Beck, 1986). Today, therapists are less likely to explain their patients' problems using drive theory, addressing the failed attachments and interpersonal difficulties that bring most people to therapy.

Limitations of the attachment model

The attachment model, for all its advantages over classical psychoanalysis, suffers from some of the same theoretical and methodological problems. The main one is that there was hardly any mention in Bowlby's books of individual differences, particularly in relation to temperament. While the model is to be commended for acknowledging the effects of natural selection on attachment behavior, it fails to consider the genetic and temperamental factors that drive individual differences. Ignoring differences in sensitivity to life events gives the mistaken impression that there is a direct relationship between early attachment patterns and adult psychopathology, which there is not.

Kagan (1998, p. 99) has also raised a question about the generalizability of the Strange Situation, which may not capture the full context of a relationship between mother and child:

> The mother and infant, who have been together for over a year, have experienced pain, pleasure, joy, and distress, and the infant's representation and behavioral reactions to the mother contain aspects of all these experiences.

Furthermore, the idea that earlier experiences are always more predictive of outcome than later ones is not consistent with the literature on child development. As Jerome Kagan (1998, p. 128) notes: "Those who favor infant determinism do not award sufficient power to the events of later childhood and adolescence".

Moreover, temperamental differences, rooted in genetic variations, affect the way that childhood experiences are processed. To make attachment theory more interactive, O'Connor et al. (2000) suggested that it could usefully be combined with behavior genetics. In longitudinal studies, Kagan (1994) has shown that differences in temperament strongly shape variations in attachment patterns, both in childhood and in adult life. Thus, heritable factors go a long way to explaining why some children with abnormal attachment patterns grow up to be normal adults, while others with secure attachment may not. Moreover, as suggested by Belsky and Pluess (2009), children who are susceptible to negative experiences in development are also more responsive to positive experiences.

Up to now, only a few studies have examined the behavior genetics of attachment, and they have not produced consistent results. One study of infants (Bokhorst et al., 2003) found little heritability in the Strange Situation, while shared environment (i.e., the effects of growing up in the same family) best accounted for disorganized attachment. However, a community study (Fearon et al., 2014) found attachment styles to be clearly heritable by that stage. Moreover, the results of longitudinal studies are mixed, with some suggesting stability over time (Waters et al., 2000), while others find that attachment patterns are not necessarily stable during childhood, and are even more unstable during adolescence (Fraley, 2002).

Another problem for attachment theory is that it retains the concept of childhood determinism in a new form, assuming that the failure of bonding between mother and child is a primary and specific cause of psychological symptoms later in life. If that were so, today's therapists might search for failed attachments in the same way that their predecessors searched for childhood trauma. Instead, it would be more accurate to say that the theory identifies one of several factors in the development of personality and psychopathology.

In short, the attachment model needs to take into account the gene-environment interactions that are so crucial in development. Again, there are no simple cause and effect relationships between childhood experiences and adult symptoms. These relationships are complex and multivariate. As pointed out by Cicchetti (2004), the same risk factors can produce many different outcomes ("multifinality"), and similar outcomes can arise from many different risks ("equifinality"). It is unfortunate that the large literature in the field of developmental psychopathology – summarized in a recent four volume book (Cicchetti, 2016) – has had so little impact on psychoanalysis.

Nonetheless, Fonagy (2001) has rightly emphasized that the rise of attachment theory built a bridge between psychoanalysis and psychology, avoiding the "splendid isolation" that characterized the past. But he is a rare analyst in having a strong scientific training, in respecting data, and in changing his ideas when new data comes in. (Twenty years ago, when Fonagy gave a talk at my department, he expressed doubts about the heritability of attachment styles; but once the evidence was available, he cheerfully changed his mind.) In recent years, Fonagy has also revised Bowlby's model (Fonagy and Allison, 2014) by focusing on what he calls the ability to have "epistemic trust" (secure attachment leading to successful social learning), as well on the capacity to "mentalize" (observing emotions in self and in others).

On the whole, research supports the concept that differences in attachment styles influence the risk for mental disorders (Cassidy and Shaver, 2015). On a statistical basis, it is better to be securely attached in childhood. But as the British child psychiatrist Michael Rutter (1995) has pointed out, there is no linear or reliably predictive relationship between childhood experiences and adult functioning. There are just too many other factors in development that matter as much or more. Attachment theory, with its emphasis on the failure of mother love, runs the risk of being still another psychoanalytic model that, by emphasizing problems in childhood, could be used to blame parents for psychopathology in their children. For example, while many clinicians have been impressed by the findings of infant research (Stern, 1985; Beebe, 2014), there is little data to suggest that observations in the first year of life can predict with any accuracy what people will be like later in life.

Applying gene-environment interaction to attachment theory is nonetheless consistent with other models. The American psychoanalyst George Engel, who was interested in the psychological factors affecting medical illnesses, developed a biopsychosocial (BPS) model that he applied to the development of mental disorders (Engel, 1980). This is another way to look at the integration, interfaces, and interactions between heritable traits, psychological phenomena, and social forces. The BPS model, which is in accord with a modern understanding of gene-environment interactions (Rutter, 2006), has been influential in psychiatry and clinical psychology.

A final limitation of Bowlby's attachment model is that it failed to consider evidence that children can have more than one primary caretaker, and that they can benefit as much from multiple attachment figures as from a mother. This mechanism, called "alloparenting" (Hrdy, 2009), makes evolutionary sense, since it protects children from the loss of a parent, as well as emotional neglect. Isolated nuclear families are not the norm in every society, while extended families provide additional psychological protection.

While the attachment model has been the subject of thousands of scientific papers, the story is not over. A recent review by Fearon and Roisman (2017) concluded that while attachment is influenced by the environment the specific determinants remain elusive, that attachment is transmitted only weakly between generations, and that attachment is not linked strongly to outcomes. The authors also note that attachment in children is not highly stable; change is the norm, not the exception.

This having been said, attachment theory is the most scientifically supported derivative of classical psychoanalysis. Yet much more research is needed to determine the multiple causes of psychopathology, of which attachment is only one piece of the puzzle.

The need for research promoting further revisions of psychoanalysis

To this day, publications about psychoanalysis almost exclusively reference other analytic articles and books. Yet there are many sub-disciplines within psychology that are highly relevant to the concerns of psychodynamic therapy, but not widely known to theorists or practitioners of psychoanalytic therapy. I have highlighted the importance of behavior genetics and developmental psychopathology. Yet at this point, neuroscience must still play a minor role, given the immaturity of the field and how little we understand about the human brain. That is likely to change over time, and analysts should be ready to welcome such insights. (Chapter 6 will describe misfires in attempts to do so on the basis of current technology and current knowledge.)

To make links with research, psychoanalysts need to show more humility. They should understand that clinical observations are only a first step in the search for truth, and that every conclusion suggested by clinical encounters needs to be converted into a hypothesis that can be tested. And constructs that cannot be studied in this way (e.g., Freud's structural model of the mind) need to be jettisoned. Moreover, failure to jettison outmoded ideas is one of the main causes of the decline of psychoanalysis. As Luyten (2015, p. 5) commented

> unless hard questions about theory and practice are questioned, orthodoxy and rigidity, already widespread in some quarters within psychoanalysis, will lead to a degenerative program of research that

will herald the downfall of psychoanalysis as an intellectual and clinical movement.

Conclusions

Overall, psychoanalysis has moved from a largely intrapsychic perspective to a model focused on problems in interpersonal relationships. However, with the exception of attachment theory, the newer models have never been empirically tested. As Eagle (2014) notes, that does not follow the procedures of science in which newer models are compared with older ones to determine if they have greater explanatory power.

Revisions to psychoanalytic theory have led us away from the 19th-century determinism that limited the thinking of Freud, and the common factor in most revisions is an increased focus on interpersonal relationships. Yet by and large, the revisions use the same epistemology, presenting a theoretical perspective, providing case examples of its application, and claiming that doing so produces better results in therapy. None of them have been tested for efficacy in clinical trials. We have no idea whether they are more effective than classical psychoanalysis, in which the evidence base is strong for brief therapy but weak for long-term, open-ended treatment.

The most impressive revision of psychoanalysis is attachment theory. However, this model has not yet been integrated into a framework that could account for wide individual differences in response to environmental challenges.

References

Ainsworth, M.D., Blehar, M.C., Waters, E., Wall, S.: *Patterns of Attachment*. Hillsdale, NJ, Erlbaum, 1978.

Beck, A.T.: *Cognitive Therapy and the Emotional Disorders*. New York, Basic Books, 1986.

Beebe, B.: My journey in infant research and psychoanalysis: Microanalysis, a social microscope. *Psychoanalytic Psychology* 2014, 31: 4–25.

Belsky, J., Pluess, M.: Beyond diathesis stress: Differential susceptibility to environmental Influences. *Psychological Bulletin* 2009, 135: 885–908.

Blanck, G., Blanck, R.: *Ego Psychology: Theory and Practice*. New York, Columbia University Press, 1994.

Bokhorst, C.L., Bakermans-Kranenburg, M.J., Fearon, P., van IJzendoorn, M.H., Fonagy, P., Schuengel, C.: The importance of shared environment in mother-infant attachment security: A behavioral genetic study. *Child Development* 2003, 74: 1769–1782.

Bowlby, J.: *Attachment and Loss*, 3 volumes. London, Hogarth Press, 1969, 1973, 1980.
Campbell, W.K., Miller, J.D., eds.: *Handbook of Narcissism and Narcissistic Personality Disorder*. New York, Wiley, 2011.
Cassidy, J., Shaver, P.R., eds.: *Handbook of Attachment: Theory, Research and Clinical Aspects*, 3rd edition. New York, Guilford Press, 2015.
Cicchetti, D.: An odyssey of discovery: Lessons learned through three decades of research on child maltreatment. *American Psychologist* 2004, 59: 4–14.
Cicchetti, D.: *Developmental Psychopathology*, 2nd edition. New York, Wiley, 2016.
Eagle, M.: *Attachment and Psychoanalysis: Theory, Research, and Clinical Implications*. New York, Guilford Press, 2014.
Edgcumbe, R.: *Anna Freud: A View of Development, Disturbance and Therapeutic Techniques*. London, Routledge, 2001.
Engel, G.L.: The clinical application of the biopsychosocial model. *American Journal of Psychiatry* 1980, 137: 535–544.
Fairbairn, W.R.: *Psychoanalytic Studies of the Personality*. London, Routledge Kegan-Paul, 1952.
Fearon, P., Schmueli-Goetz, Y., Viding, E., Fonagy, P., Plomin, R.: Genetic and environmental influences on adolescent attachment. *Journal of Child Psychology and Psychiatry* 2014, 5: 1033–1041.
Fearon, R.M.P., Roisman, G.I.: Attachment theory: Progress and future directions. *Current Opinion in Psychology* 2017, 15: 131–136.
Fisher, S., Greenberg, R.P.: *Freud Scientifically Reappraised*. New York, Wiley, 1996.
Fonagy, P.: *Attachment Theory and Psychoanalysis*. New York, Other Press, 2001.
Fonagy, P., Allison, E.: The role of mentalization and epistemic trust in the therapeutic relationship. *Psychotherapy* 2014, 31: 372–380.
Fonagy, P., Campbell, C.: Bad blood revisited: Attachment and psychoanalysis. *British Journal of Psychiatry* 2015, 31: 229–250.
Fraley, R.C.: Attachment stability from infancy to adulthood: Meta-analysis and dynamic modeling of developmental mechanisms. *Personality and Social Psychology* 2002, 6: 123–151.
Fromm, E.: *Escape from Freedom*. New York, Fawcett, 1940/1978.
Goldberg, A.: *The Prison House of Psychoanalysis*. Hillsdale, NJ, Analytic Press, 1990.
Greenberg, J., Mitchell, S.: *Object Relations in Psychoanalytic Theory*. Cambridge, MA, Harvard University Press, 1983.
Grosskurth, P.: *Melanie Klein: Her World and Her Work*. New York, Knopf, 1984.
Guntrip, H.: *Schizoid Phenomena, Object Relations, and the Self*. New York, International Universities Press, 1969.
Harlow, H.: The nature of love. *American Psychologist* 1958, 13: 673–685.
Holmes, J.: *John Bowlby and Attachment Theory*, 2nd edition. London, Routledge, 2014.
Horney, K.: *The Neurotic Personality of Our Time*. New York, Norton, 1940.
Hrdy, S.B.: *Mothers and Others: The Evolutionary Origins of Mutual Understanding*. Cambridge, Harvard University Press, 2009.
Kagan, J.L.: *Galen's Prophecy: Temperament in Human Nature*. New York, Basic Books, 1994.
Kagan, J.L.: *Three Seductive Ideas*. Cambridge, MA, Harvard University Press, 1998.
Kohut, H.: *The Analysis of the Self*. New York, International Universities Press, 1970.
Linehan, M.M.: *Cognitive-Behavioral Treatment of Borderline Personality Disorder*. New York, Guilford Press, 1993.

Luyten, P.: Unholy questions about five central tenets of psychoanalysis that need to be empirically verified. *Psychoanalytic Inquiry* 2015, 35: 5–23.

Main, M., Hesse, E., Goldwyn, R.: Studying differences in language usage in recounting attachment history: An introduction to the AAI. In H. Steele, M. Steele, eds.: *Clinical Applications of the Adult Attachment Interview*. New York, Guilford Press, 2008, pp. 31–68.

Mills, J.: A critique of relational psychoanalysis. *Psychoanalytic Psychol*ogy 2005, 22: 165–188.

Mills, J.: *Conundrums: A Critique of Contemporary Psychoanalysis*. New York, Taylor & Francis, 2012.

O'Connor, T.G., Croft, C., Steele, H.: The contributions of behavioural genetic studies to attachment theory. *Attachment & Human Development* 2000, 2: 107–122.

Rogers, C.: *Counseling and Psychotherapy: Newer Concepts in Practice*. New York, Houghton Mifflin, 1942.

Rutter, M.J.: Clinical implications of attachment concepts: Retrospect and prospect. *Journal of Child Psychology and Psychiatry* 1995, 36: 549–571.

Rutter, M.K.: *Genes and Behavior: Nature-Nurture Interplay Explained*. London, Blackwell, 2006.

Stern, D.: *The Interpersonal World of the Infant*. New York, Basic Books, 1985.

Sullivan, H.: *The Interpersonal Theory of Psychiatry*. New York, Norton, 1953.

Truax, C., Carkhuff, R.: *Toward Effective Counseling and Psychotherapy: Training and Practice*. Chicago, Aldine, 1967.

Waters, E., Merrick, S., Treboux, D., Crowell, J., Albersheim, L.: Attachment security from infancy to early adulthood: A 20-year longitudinal study. *Child Development* 2000, 71: 684–689.

Winnicott, D.W.: *Collected Papers*. London, Tavistock, 1958.

Chapter 4

The road to integration

The price of intellectual isolation

Psychoanalysis has hurt itself through its preference for intellectual isolation. Separation from science has led to a failure to find bridges to mainstream psychology or psychiatry. Within the walls of its institutes, practitioners who hold the same beliefs can find validation, but not always new ideas. In the absence of a research culture, ideas are held out of respect for tradition. Thus free-standing institutes tend to become echo chambers, in which one's point of view is not likely to be seriously challenged. This situation stands in contrast to science, in which almost every idea, no matter how dearly held, undergoes constant criticism. The same principle applies to reigning paradigms (Kuhn, 1962). Progress in science is marked by the overturning of theories, even if they have survived for decades, or even centuries.

Psychoanalysis, like any other discipline aspiring to find the truth, belongs in the university, where scholars and researchers with different backgrounds work together (Wallerstein, 2011). Otto Kernberg (2000, 2011) has severely criticized the insularity of analytic training, particularly the fact that candidates are never taught research skills, or even to think like scientists. Kernberg has a long history of collaboration with researchers, and wrote up quantitative data on the results of psychoanalytic treatment at the Menninger Clinic (Kernberg et al., 1972). He was also involved in developing Transference Focused Psychotherapy (TFP), a treatment for borderline personality disorder that has undergone clinical testing (Clarkin et al., 2007).

While analysts who hold academic positions are more likely to be interested in research, most institutes have remained separate from universities, and many members function as solo practitioners. There are some notable exceptions: among the most prominent are the Columbia University Center for Psychoanalytic Training and Research in New York, the Psychoanalysis Unit at University College, London, and the Menninger Hospital associated with Baylor University in Houston. Thus, while free-standing institutes continue to require all candidates to master the complete works of Freud, those that are nested in universities are more open to new points of view.

As the British philosopher Michael Lacewing (2013) has suggested, psychoanalysis has not, up to now, functioned as a science, but it could and it should. Only a few practicing analysts have sufficient training to carry out research. They lack contact with university settings that provide opportunities for clinicians and researchers to pool resources, and to search for connections between clinical data and empirical testing of hypotheses. Unfortunately, that does not happen very often. What is needed is a commitment to empiricism, and an openness to changing theory and practice in the light of research. Instead of asking candidates and practitioners to adopt a "psychoanalytic perspective", openness to different perspectives that can modify the paradigm need to be introduced.

The future of psychoanalytic research

Fonagy (2004, p. 78) has proposed the following agenda for an integration of psychoanalysis into psychiatry and clinical psychology:

> In order to ensure a future for psychoanalysis and psychoanalytic therapies within psychiatry, psychoanalytic practitioners must change their attitude in the direction of a more systematic outlook. This attitude shift would be characterized by several components: a) The evidence base of psychoanalysis should be strengthened by adopting additional data-gathering methods that are now widely available in biological and social science. New evidence may assist psychoanalysts in resolving theoretical differences, a feat which the current database of predominantly anecdotal clinical accounts have not been capable of achieving. b) The logic of psychoanalytic discourse would need to change from its overdependence on rhetoric and global constructs to using specific constructs that allow for cumulative data-gathering. c) Flaws in psychoanalytic scientific reasoning, such as failures to consider alternative accounts for observations (beyond that favored by the

author), should be overcome and in particular, the issue of genetic and social influence should be approached with increased sophistication. d) The isolation of psychoanalysis should be replaced by active collaboration with other mental health disciplines.

Fonagy's emphasis on changing attitudes is very much in concord with the thrust of this book. But what sort of active collaboration with other disciplines is needed? As discussed in Chapter 2, the essential elements of psychoanalytic theory remain open for further evaluation using empirical methods. Let us consider some of the principal issues discussed in Chapter 1.

The unconscious mind

Cognitive science supports the importance of unconscious mechanisms in thought, emotion, and behavior. At this point, research is not needed to prove their existence. Yet we cannot know what lies in the unconscious without a way of measuring its contents. Clinical methods are ultimately little more than educated guesses that can be biased by theoretical preconceptions.

There are now several research methods for evaluating unconscious mechanisms. One of the most fertile has been the study of subliminal perception, in which words or pictures are flashed on a screen too rapidly to reach conscious awareness (Augusto, 2010). Another is cueing, in which the presentation of one set of words or images affects the way a later set is perceived (Posner, 1980). A third is the measurement of defense mechanisms using validated scales (Bond, 2004). A fourth is research on hypnosis (Oakley and Halligan, 2013). A fifth is research on behavioral economics – to be discussed in Chapter 9 (Kahnemann, 2011).

In recent years, there has also been interest in studying the unconscious using the technology of brain imaging (Berlin and Koch, 2009). However, as Chapter 6 will show, current studies of his complex relationship have been vastly over-hyped. Neuroscience must advance much further first. And that is a project not for a decade, but for a century. Consciousness, as well as unconscious processes such as many emotions, will eventually be linked to neural connections. But as Chapter 6 will discuss, current theories based on connectionism (e.g., Cuthbert and Insel, 2013) suffer from being both vague and naïve. This having been said, we will probably understand the unconscious better in the future.

Memory

Memory research has not found strong evidence for a process of repression, at least in the sense that Freud originally proposed (Bower, 1990). As discussed in Chapter 2, the mind is not a tape recorder, but a highly selective system for keeping track of what we most need to remember. At the same time, memory functions as a way of processing live events and modifying them as individuals are exposed to newer experiences (Richards and Frankland, 2017). Moreover, every time we access a memory, we revise and change it.

What research does support is a concept of "repressive coping", a personality style associated with not thinking about painful things in life (Furnham and Lay, 2016). But that pattern more closely resembles suppression (conscious forgetting) than repression.

Childhood experiences and adult psychopathology

Research fails to support a simple causal relationship between experiences in childhood and mental disorders in adulthood (Paris, 2000). On the other hand, there is massive data supporting the conclusion that adverse experiences in childhood are *risk factors* for psychopathology (Rutter, 2006). The mistake has been a failure to distinguish risk factors (which make pathology more likely on a statistical basis) and causes that predictably lead to specific symptoms or life problems.

This Gordian knot can be untied by viewing causality as multivariate, not univariate. In other words, research on the effects of childhood experience needs to combine biological factors (genes, neurocircuitry, neurotransmitters) with psychological factors (trauma, neglect, dysfunctional families), as well as social factors (poverty, rapid social change). This paradigm shift leads to a much more complex model that is ultimately more valid. It also suggests that child development research has to be conducted from multiple perspectives that have been shown to interact with each other.

Psychoanalysis, neurobiology, and behavior genetics

We should not expect to find neural correlates (measured by fMRI and other neurobiological methods) of constructs proposed by Freud or by other analysts, all of which was introduced at a time when this research had not even begun. This is why Kandel (1998) was wrong in suggesting that neuroscience will be able to map Freud's theories onto brain anatomy. "Cherry-picking" neuroscience to confirm Freud's ideas is simplistic. Localization of mental constructs is limited by the complexity or the relationship between highly interactive neural circuits and observable behaviors thoughts, and emotions. Yet (as Chapter 6 will show) while "neuropsychoanalysis" (Panskepp and Solms, 2012) is a misfire, a more detailed understanding of the complexities of the brain should eventually have relevance to clinical work.

One line of research that could be more fruitful is a research program on psychodynamic constructs that takes heritable temperamental variations into account, using data from behavioral genetics. This point of view has applications to practice. It is not scientifically valid to tell patients that their present problems are almost entirely driven by life experiences. One of the most obvious facts that disconfirms this assumption is that siblings growing up in the same family are no more similar than if they were strangers (Harris, 1998). In a previous book (Paris, 1998), I suggested that interpretations of the past in psychotherapy could usefully be framed by a statement along the following lines: "given your inborn sensitivity, it is understandable that you reacted to life events in a different way from other members of your family".

Fonagy (2003, p. 234) pointed out how behavioral genetics leads to a different and much more complex model of child development:

> It is probably true that we have previously exaggerated the importance of parents for development: adoption studies, in particular, show that much of parental influence is illusory. It is likely that personality characteristics in the child which have been thought of as a reaction to the parents' behavior, are in fact genetic predispositions. The personality trait and the associated form of parenting (criticism, warmth, or even abuse) are both consequences of the same genes in the parent and the child. Equally, adoption studies suggest that children with genetic tendencies toward – for instance – aggression will elicit more hostile and coercive parenting.

Again, research requires the use of multivariate models, with each risk factor, from biology, psychology, or society, having cumulative and interactive effects. Here psychoanalysis, with its emphasis on subjective experiences, has something to contribute. One need not assume that the "narrative truth" of individual perspectives on experience correspond to "historical truth" (Spence, 1982). Rather, people react differently to life experiences, depending on their temperament (Rutter, 2006). People also differ in how sensitive they are to their environment, good or bad (Belsky and Pluess, 2009). Thus, some children do better than average in a good environment, and worse than average in a bad one. It is possible that some of these variations in sensitivity are rooted in neurobiology. In a famous study of a birth cohort of children followed up into adulthood, Caspi et al. (2003) hypothesized that environmental sensitivity could be related to a gene for the serotonin transporter. While that explanation is too simple, this paper, which underlines the interactions between life events and temperament, is one of the most quoted papers in the history of psychology.

In short, no univariate model of child development or of psychopathology can ever be valid. Biological psychiatry has often made the mistake of ignoring the environment in favor of genes, neurotransmitters, and neural connections. Psychoanalysis has made the mistake of ignoring the biological factors that underlie individual variations in response to stressful environments.

Efficacy of psychoanalytic psychotherapy

To address this crucial issue, two lines of research are needed. While brief psychodynamic psychotherapy is clearly efficacious, we need better studies of *how* that treatment helps patients. Luborsky et al. (1994) had hypothesized that if therapists correctly identify and focus on a psychodynamic theme (which they call the Core Conflict Relationship Theme or CCRT), then therapy is more likely to move forward. However, that conclusion is not well supported by research showing that psychodynamic therapy is as effective as CBT (Gibbons et al., 2016), and that all therapies work through common mechanisms (Wampold, 2001).

In this light, it seems necessary to question whether or not interpretations of past events and transference phenomena are as crucial to outcome as analysts have claimed. As Spence (1982) once suggested, therapy is a narrative procedure that makes sense of life experience, even if its explanations need not be literally true.

The second issue concerns whether long-term psychoanalysis or psychoanalytic therapy is necessary uniquely effective for some patients. Studying this subject properly would be enormously expensive. One can imagine an ideal study of a large sample in a randomized controlled trial, but the cost would be in the millions of dollars, so this kind of study will not happen anytime soon. Yet until we have more data, we should be cautious about directing our patients to the most resource-intensive options.

In summary, there are many questions for which psychoanalytic theory and practice provide important hypotheses to be tested. There are also many problems in psychology which could benefit from a psychodynamic perspective. But that can only happen if the bridge to psychology is actually built. And for it to happen, we need leadership from influential psychoanalysts, who must be open to change and promote joining the scientific community.

Integration in psychoanalysis and psychotherapy

Psychoanalysis, since the time of Freud, has believed its methods to be "pure gold", with practical adaptations seen as "copper" (Freud, 1919). But research on the outcome of psychoanalytic therapy, while encouraging in some ways, has never supported the primacy of psychodynamic methods over CBT or other competitors.

Instead, psychoanalysts can take pride in the fact that most other forms of psychotherapy make much use of ideas derived from the classical model. There are differences between CBT and psychodynamic therapy in that cognitive therapy structures treatment sessions, gives out homework, and does not hesitate to give advice. However, it may not be the case that psychoanalysts do none of those things. It is a question of emphasis. For example, one evidence-based treatment, interpersonal psychotherapy (IPT; Weissman et al., 2007), might be described as psychodynamic therapy without the past. It also resembles CBT. Thus IPT, like relational psychoanalysis, focuses on problems in current intimate relationships, which of course are the usual reason for seeking therapy in the first place.

While there are hundreds of named psychotherapies, they are all variations on the themes developed by psychodynamic and cognitive therapy. The movement for *psychotherapy integration* aims to meld together the best ideas from all sources, creating a single form of psychotherapy (Norcross and Goldfried, 2005). This concept is highly consistent with empirical evidence. There is no reason why psychoanalysts cannot make use of cognitive interventions, and there is no reason why CBT therapists cannot make use of ideas derived from psychoanalysis.

Psychotherapy has greatly suffered from the existence of multiple schools of thought, many of which are identified by a catchy acronym. To consider one example, Eye Movement Desensitization and Reprocessing (EMDR) for post-traumatic stress disorder, while cleverly marketed, has much the same outcome as CBT, and differs only in its idiosyncratic use of eye movements (Seidler and Wagner, 2006). There is little need for so many competing psychotherapies, few of which are based on data. Instead, proponents invoke prestige of the founder and present case histories. But that is not evidence-based therapy, but *eminence-based* therapy, or *acronym-based* therapy.

A single form of psychotherapy would be a mélange of psychodynamic and cognitive methods. But it would draw strongly on the analytic tradition of understanding life histories. This is not to say that interpretations linking past and present are, by themselves, "mutative". While there is little research in this area, it is often useful to point out to patients how they are repeating their early experiences with their family in current relationships. This having been said, patients still need to work to change these patterns. In psychoanalysis, the length of therapy is often attributed to a need to "work through" such difficulties. However, there is no reason why patients cannot do this work after therapy, or during periods when therapy is suspended (Alexander and French, 1946).

We can also consider why the place of transference interpretation in an integrated psychotherapy can at best be described as uncertain. Other forms of psychotherapy, particularly CBT, are effective without using transference interpretation. It is not part of the common factors that drive positive outcomes. Moreover, the evidence that these techniques are essential for good results is at best mixed (Høglend and Gabbard, 2012). Some research has supported the use of transference interventions (Malan, 1980), but others have found negative effects (Piper et al., 1991), possibly related to misguided attempts to deal with negative reactions in patients by interpretation alone. This is not to say that *observing* transference (and counter-transference) is not useful, but to state that it may not play the crucial role in the therapeutic process often attributed to it.

An integrated psychotherapy would put most emphasis on the *common factors* that make psychotherapy work. These factors were first described over 80 years ago by the psychologist Saul Rosenzweig (1936): (a) the inspiring or stimulating aspects of the therapist's personality, (b) the reintegration of personality through the systematic application of some therapeutic ideology, (c) implicit psychological processes such as catharsis or social reconditioning, and (d) the reformulation of psychological events. A more radical formulation was proposed by Jerome Frank, who attributed recovery in psychotherapy to the recovery of morale (Frank and Frank, 1991). While Frank's concept is too simple, it remains true that research does not support the importance of specific over non-specific interventions (Duncan et al., 2010).

Thus, research provides support for the use of interventions derived from other forms of treatment as part of psychodynamically oriented therapy. An integrated psychotherapy, i.e., a single model of treatment rather than one focused on a single theory, can offer many advantages. An integrated approach has been shown to be effective for patients with a wide range of psychopathology (Norcross and Goldfried, 2005).

Decades ago, Wachtel (1975) proposed combining psychodynamic and behavioral interventions into one form of therapy. Later, Safran and Segal (1995) pointed out that since CBT also deals with many interpersonal problems, there can be a strong convergence between cognitive and psychodynamic methods. As Bateman (2002, p. 19) pointed out:

> Further integration of psychotherapies will only come about if we identify more precisely the mechanisms of therapeutic change. It is not just a case of picking a bit of this and a bit of that. Once mediators of change are established we will need to rebuild our cherished theories, and decide on the sequencing of interventions and on whom the interventions are to be carried out. If psychoanalysis and cognitive-behaviour therapy are to remain vibrant and living disciplines they must open themselves up to each other and change according to new findings of process research.

In summary, psychoanalytic theory and practice have not thus far been well researched, but certainly could be (Westen, 1998). The convergence of different disciplines has greatly advanced many branches of science (Watson, 2015). As a discipline, psychoanalysis could benefit from moving outside its paradigm, and learning from behavioral genetics, neurobiology, developmental psychology, and cognitive science.

References

Alexander, F., French, T.: *Psychoanalytic Therapy*. New York, Ronald Press, 1946.

Augusto, L.M.: Unconscious knowledge: A survey. *Advances in Cognitive Psychology* 2010, 6: 116–141.

Bateman, A.: Integrative therapy from an analytic perspective. In J. Holmes, A. Bateman: *Integration in Psychotherapy: Models and Methods*. Oxford, Oxford University Press, 2002, pp. 11–25.

Belsky, J., Pluess, M.: Beyond diathesis Stress: Differential susceptibility to environmental influences. *Psychological Bulletin* 2009, 135: 885–908.

Berlin, H.A., Koch, C.: Neuroscience meets psychoanalysis. *Scientific American Mind* 2009: 16–19.

Bond, M.: Empirical studies of defense style: Relationships with psychopathology and change. *Harvard Review of Psychiatry* 2004, 12: 263–278.

Bower, G.H.: Awareness, the unconscious, and repression. In J. Singer, ed.: *Repression and Dissociation*. Chicago, University of Chicago Press, 1990, pp. 209–231.

Caspi, A., Sugden, K., Moffitt, T.E., Taylor, A., Craig, W., Harrington, H.: Influence of life stress on depression: Moderation by a polymorphism in the 5-HTT gene. *Science* 2003, 301: 386–389.

Clarkin, J.F., Levy, K.N., Lenzenweger, M.F., Kernberg, O.F.: Evaluating three treatments for borderline personality disorder: A multiwave study. *American Journal of Psychiatry* 2007, 164: 1–8.

Cuthbert, B.N., Insel, T.R.: Toward the future of psychiatric diagnosis: The seven pillars of RDoC. *BMC Medicine* 2013, 11: 126.

Duncan, B.L., Miller, S.D., Wampold, B.E., Hubble, M.A., eds.: *The Heart and Soul of Change: Delivering What Works in Therapy*, 2nd edition. Washington, DC, American Psychological Association, 2010.

Fonagy, P.: Genetics, developmental psychopathology, and psychoanalytic theory: The case for ending our (not so) splendid isolation. *Psychoanalytic Inquiry* 2003, 23: 218–247.

Fonagy, P.: Psychoanalysis today. *World Psychiatry* 2004, 2: 73–80.

Frank, J.D., Frank, J.B.: *Persuasion and Healing*, 3rd edition. Baltimore, Johns Hopkins Press, 1991.

Freud, S.: Lines of advance in psycho-analytic therapy. In J. Strachey, ed.: *Standard Edition of the Complete Works of Sigmund Freud*, Volume 17, Hogarth Press, 1959, pp. 157–168 (first published 1919).

Furnham, A., Lay, A.: Repressive coping and theories about psychotherapy. *Journal of Psychology and Psychotherapy* 2016, 6: 283–293.

Gibbons, M.B.C., Gallop, R., Thompson, D.: Comparative effectiveness of cognitive therapy and dynamic psychotherapy for major depressive disorder in a community mental health setting: A randomized clinical non-inferiority trial. *JAMA Psychiatry* 2016, 73: 904–912.

Harris, J.R.: *The Nurture Assumption*. New York, Free Press, 1998.

Høglend, P., Gabbard, G.O.: When is transference work useful in psychodynamic psychotherapy? A review of empirical research. In R. Levy, J. Ablon, H. Kächele, eds.: *Psychodynamic Psychotherapy Research, Current Clinical Psychiatry Series*. Totowa, NJ, Humana Press, 2012, pp. 449–467.

Kahnemann, D.: *Thinking Fast and Slow*. New York, Palgrave MacMillan, 2011.

Kandel, E.: A new intellectual framework for psychiatry. *American Journal of Psychiatry* 1998, 155: 457–469.
Kernberg, O.F.: A concerned critique of psychoanalytic education. *International Journal of Psychoanalysis* 2000, 81: 97–107.
Kernberg, O.F.: Psychoanalysis and the university: A difficult relationship. *International Journal of Psychoanalysis* 2011, 92: 609–622.
Kernberg, O.F., Coyne, L., Appelbaum, A., Horwitz, L., Voth, H.: Final report of the Menninger Psychotherapy Research Project. *Bulletin of the Menninger Clinic* 1972, 36: 1–275.
Kuhn, T.: *The Structure of Scientific Revolutions*. Chicago, University of Chicago Press, 1962.
Lacewing, M.: Could psychoanalysis be a science? In K.W.M. Fulford, M. Davies, J. Sadler, G. Stanghellini, T. Thornton, eds.: *The Oxford Handbook of Philosophy and Psychiatry*. New York, Oxford University Press, 2013, pp. 3–41.
Lazar, S.G.: The cost-effectiveness of psychotherapy for the major psychiatric diagnoses. *Psychodynamic Psychiatry* 2014, 42: 423–457.
Luborsky, L., Popp, C., Luborsky, E., Mark, D.: The core conflictual relationship theme. *Psychotherapy Research* 1994, 4: 172–183.
Malan, D.: *A Study of Brief Psychotherapy*. London, Springer, 1980.
Norcross, J.C., Goldfried, M.R.: *Handbook of Psychotherapy Integration*, 2nd edition. New York, Oxford University Press, 2005.
Oakley, D.A., Halligan, P.W.: Hypnotic suggestion: Opportunities for cognitive neuroscience. *Nature Reviews Neuroscience* 2013, 14 (8): 565–576.
Panskepp, J., Solms, M.: What is neuropsychoanalysis? Clinically relevant studies of the minded brain. *Trends in Cognitive Sciences* 2012, 16: 6–8.
Paris, J.: *Nature and Nurture in Psychiatry*. Washington, DC, American Psychiatric Publishing, 1998.
Paris, J.: *Myths of Childhood*. New York, Taylor & Francis, 2000.
Piper, W.E., Azim, H.F., Joyce, A.S., McCallum, M.: Transference interpretations, therapeutic alliance, and outcome in short-term individual psychotherapy. *Archives of General Psychiatry* 1991, 48: 946–953.
Posner, M.I.: Orienting of attention. *Quarterly Journal of Experimental Psychology* 1980, 32: 3–25.
Richards, B.A., Frankland, P.W.: The persistence and transience of memory. *Neuron* 2017, 94: 1072–1084.
Rosenzweig, S.: Some implicit common factors in diverse methods of psychotherapy: "At last the Dodo said, 'Everybody has won and all must have prizes'". *American Journal of Orthopsychiatry* 1936, 6: 412–415.
Rutter, M.: *Genes and Behavior: Nature-Nurture Interplay Explained*. London, Blackwell, 2006.
Safran, J., Segal, Z.: *Interpersonal Process in Cognitive Therapy*. Mahwah, NJ, Jason Aronson, 1995.
Schacter, D.: *Searching for Memory: The Brain, the Mind, and the Past*. New York, Basic Books, 1995.
Seidler, G.H., Wagner, F.E.: Comparing the efficacy of EMDR and trauma-focused cognitive-behavioral therapy in the treatment of PTSD: A meta-analytic study. *Psychological Medicine* 2006, 36: 1515–152.
Spence, D.: *Narrative Truth and Historical Truth*. New York, Norton, 1982.

Wachtel, P.: *Psychoanalysis and Behavior Therapy: Toward an Integration*. New York, Basic Books, 1975.

Wallerstein, R.: Psychoanalysis in the university: The natural home for education and research. *International Journal of Psychoanalysis* 2011, 92: 623–639.

Wampold, B.E.: *The Great Psychotherapy Debate: Models, Methods, and Findings*. Mahwah, NJ, Erlbaum Associates, 2001.

Watson, P.: *Convergence: The Idea at the Heart of Science*. New York, Simon and Schuster, 2015.

Weissman, M.M., Markowitz, J.C., Klerman, G.L.: *Clinician's Quick Guide to Interpersonal Psychotherapy*. New York, Oxford University Press, 2007.

Westen, D.: The scientific legacy of Sigmund Freud: Towards a psychodynamically informed psychological science. *Psychological Bulletin* 1998, 124: 128–136.

Chapter 5

Making treatment brief and accessible

Problems in access to treatment

Mental disorders are very common. Nearly half of the population will meet criteria for at least one of the conditions defined in diagnostic manuals within any given year (Kessler et al., 2005). Even if we were to exclude minor and transient conditions, these numbers constitute a major public health challenge. The diagnoses that affect most people (anxiety, depression, personality disorder, substance abuse) are all treatable with psychotherapy.

Yet the needs of the population for evidence-based psychological treatment are not currently being met. Psychiatrists are prescribing more drugs and spending less time with patients (Olfson et al., 2002; Olfson and Marcus, 2010). Psychologists, who now provide most courses of psychotherapy, sometimes carry out generic treatments that are insufficiently specific, especially for severe psychopathology. Social workers who practice psychotherapy in institutions carry heavy caseloads, and may lack sufficient training to carry "heavier" patients.

The goal of providing psychotherapy to meet needs in the clinical population is constricted by limited human resources. Even a dramatic increase in mental health workers would not address these population needs. Measures have been taken in the UK to fund psychotherapy within the National Health Service, and to conduct systematic evaluations on its effectiveness (Goldbeck-Wood, 2004). Although therapy under this Improving Access to Psychological Therapies (IAPT) program has reached nearly a million people (Clark, 2018), the numbers are still insufficient to meet the needs of the larger community. But what is particularly positive about this initiative is that it is national, publically funded, accountable, and is conducting large-scale research into its efficacy. And while the focus has been on CBT, Peter Fonagy has been a consultant in applying this approach to child and adolescent services.

In contrast, therapies, particularly in North America, are provided by mental health systems that can barely be called systematic. The length of therapy is driven not by clinical evaluations, but by private insurance. Moreover, when therapies are lengthy, they will not be insured. Thus classical psychoanalysis (or even once a week psychodynamic therapy over several years), are only available to the wealthy. If we assume a fee of $150 an hour, people with limited incomes would still have to struggle to pay for therapy lasting as little as a few months.

The relative unavailability of psychotherapy is a tragic situation, especially given the strong evidence base demonstrating its efficacy and effectiveness (Lambert, 2013). Once again, the very large body of research on psychotherapy outcome is based almost entirely on treatments that last for a few months. We have no evidence to support offering long-term therapy on a routine basis. There is also no evidence that seeing patients more than once a week provides better results.

Some defenders of traditional models have quoted a study by Seligman (1995), which surveyed readers of Consumers Report on their experiences in therapy. It is probable that a large percentage of these consumers, surveyed 25 years ago, received psychodynamic therapy. One of the findings was that most felt longer treatment was preferable. But this was an unusual sample of educated people who could either afford therapy or who had good insurance. The survey also lacked a control group. Again, we have almost no efficacy data (i.e., RCTs) on therapies that last for a year or more. The results of clinical trials that have found that therapies lasting for a few months are efficacious cannot be generalized to long-term treatments like psychoanalysis. From the point of view of research, extended therapies remain *terra incognita*. But while short-term therapies should be a default, longer treatment may still have a place in the mental health system.

Access to psychotherapy

Let us examine what survey data tell us about the provision of psychotherapy, particularly in the US, where this issue has been the subject of research. The most extensive study, limited to psychiatrists, was conducted by two researchers at Columbia University, Mark Olfson and

Steven Marcus (2010), and it showed an overall decline in usage. The findings showed that in 2007 about 3% of the population received talking therapy, a figure that remained stable over a ten-year period. However, the use of psychotherapy *only* (as opposed to being combined with medication) went down from about 16% to less than 11%. The mean number of annual visits per patient declined from 9.7 to 7.9. This number falls below what research shows most patients minimally require, i.e. 10–20 sessions (Howard et al., 1986). The mean expenditure per visit in 2007 was $95 (a figure that would be much higher today).

Most therapists use short-term therapy on a regular basis. As long as 20 years ago, Levenson and Davidovitz (2000) found that 89% of psychologists were offering brief treatment, and, on average, spent about half their time doing so. But is this level of service meeting the needs of the population? The question is crucial, given that the disorders that are most prevalent in the population (depression, anxiety, personality disorders, substance use) are also those that are usually targeted by psychological methods.

Yet a survey of consumers (Chamberlin, 2004) found that only 70% of the population considers mental health care access to be adequate. A more recent report by the Substance Abuse and Mental Health Administration (Han et al., 2015, p. 1) reported: "Nearly half of the 5.3 million American adults who perceived the need for, but did not receive mental health care, reported they did not receive it because they could not afford the cost of it. A total of 11.8 million Americans reported that they had an unmet need for additional mental health services". This conclusion was replicated in a later survey (Substance Abuse and Mental Health Administration, 2015).

Thus, given the high rate of mental disorders in the community, mental health services are only fully accessible to those with good financial resources. There can be little doubt that if psychotherapy were better insured, there would be a strong demand for places in the practices of currently active clinicians. But that change alone would not solve the problem. The currently unmet demand for treatment would be strong enough to fill practices and clinics.

Yet as long as psychotherapy is lengthy, most therapists would have a waiting list that would still be a serious barrier to accessibility. And when therapy is lengthy, the system becomes blocked and slots do not often open for new patients. This was the experience for psychiatrists in the Canadian system after being fully insured by governments in 1970 (Paris, 2016).

The mental health sector is poorly funded and poorly insured. On top of that, administrators who make decisions tend to have a bias against psychotherapy, both in terms of efficacy and cost-effectiveness. They are generally unaware of the well supported finding that insuring even a few months of therapy a year saves money, by reducing hospitalizations, emergency room visits, and a need for unemployment benefits (Lazar, 2014). A recent meta-analysis showed that about 75% of patients seeking mental health treatment prefer psychotherapy over pharmacotherapy (McHugh et al., 2013).

Still, the unanswered question is whether long-term therapy can accomplish things that short-term treatment cannot. I cannot dismiss this option, but consider it applicable only to the minority of those seeking therapy. I have worked with many patients over periods of about two years, and my own personality disorder clinics, while considering brief therapy to be a default condition, offers selected patients 18–24 months of therapy. But these patients are in the minority (Laporte et al., 2018).

As reviewed in Chapter 2, the scientific evidence for long-term therapy remains weak. Moreover, most patients looking for mental health treatment prefer brief therapy (Hemmings, 2000). The problem is that they cannot afford it. And even with lower cost treatment, they may not be able to find it.

The evidence supporting brief psychotherapy

Psychotherapy is an evidence-based treatment with a strong base in research (Luborsky and Luborsky, 2006; Lambert, 2013). The good news from randomized controlled trials is that all forms of psychotherapy produce results in most patients within a few months (Lambert, 2013). Thus, brief psychodynamic therapy is as efficacious as other methods, including CBT, and it also compares well to courses of antidepressants. Based on systematic reviews and meta-analyses of clinical trials comparing the outcome of psychodynamic therapy to other forms of treatment (Gerber et al., 2011; Abbass et al., 2012; Cuijpers et al., 2008; Steinert et al., 2017), we can conclude that this treatment is as efficacious as either CBT or medication for depression and anxiety (i.e., for most of the patients that clinicians see).

It is not widely understood that virtually all empirical studies concern brief treatment, while therapy lasting for more than a year remains unstudied or unsupported. The findings of research on brief therapy cannot be generalized to long-term treatments such as classical psychoanalysis. Yet therapy has a tendency to continue beyond a year with or without an evidence base to support doing so. Patients who have enough money or insurance coverage can continue seeing therapists indefinitely.

The issue here is *accountability*. Nowadays this principle is an expectation for practice of all kinds, clinical psychology, social work, or in medicine. But in psychotherapy there is no broadly accepted system to make practice accountable, and to regulate the provision of psychotherapy in terms of outcome or cost-benefit (Johnson, 1996; Eagle, 2011).

Unfortunately, empirical findings are not always integrated into clinical practice. As discussed in Chapter 2, studies examining the outcome of long-term psychodynamic therapy are not convincing, since they are almost uniformly pre-post comparisons without controls. Reporting a recent meta-analysis of randomized and quasi-randomized trials of long-term psychoanalytic psychotherapy (LTPP), Smit et al. (2012, p. 81) concluded:

> the recovery rate of various mental disorders was equal after LTPP or various control treatments, including treatment as usual. The effect sizes of the individual trials varied substantially in direction and magnitude. In contrast to previous reviews, we found the evidence for the effectiveness of LTPP to be limited and at best conflicting.

These conclusions are also in concordance with one of the most consistent findings in psychotherapy research: that most forms of treatment, whatever their theoretical basis, tend to yield similar outcomes (Wampold, 2001). This equivalence between therapies raises questions about whether specific techniques, either psychodynamic interpretations or CBT-derived tools, are the key element in producing a successful outcome. Does it really make a difference whether transference interpretations or CBT homework make a difference in success? We do not really know. It seems likely that any therapy that solves problems in interpersonal relationships is likely to be helpful.

Given the strong evidence for brief therapy, and the absence of good evidence for long-term therapy, brief forms of psychodynamic psychotherapy, with 10–20 sessions once a week, should be one of the major options for clinicians in the treatment of common mental disorders. This model would offer effective treatment available to a larger population, and would be in accord with the findings of psychotherapy research. Moreover, most patients in practice who undergo psychotherapy have only a brief course of treatment, usually by mutual agreement with the therapist.

A modification that has been recommended for brief psychodynamic therapy is to identify a *focus* for therapy and to follow the same theme in every session (Summers and Barber, 2012). This concept was first developed by the British psychoanalyst David Malan (1980), who conducted some of the first research showing that brief therapy usually works. Following a focus can make treatment more coherent and targeted. Classical versions of psychoanalytic therapy, offering frequent sessions over several years, tend to be lacking in this regard, and run the danger of becoming diffuse and untargeted. Brief therapies, with time limits, can limit regression and encourage work on specific current problems.

One of the more interesting concepts behind brief therapy is to see time limits not as a problem, but an opportunity. That was the idea behind *time-limited psychotherapy*, developed in the 1970s by the American psychoanalyst James Mann (1980), who wrote eloquently about the relation of time to the human life span. In his model, a time limit is essential to promoting psychological development and forward movement. Wanting to stay longer in therapy can be seen as a resistance to addressing developmental tasks. Thus, therapy is limited to 12 sessions – which also happens to be close to the typical length (10–20 sessions) that research shows to be consistently effective (Howard et al., 1986).

I vividly remember seeing James Mann presenting at a 1977 conference. He surprised me by using a case referred from the emergency room, in which a working-class man had threatened to kill himself and his wife. In spite of this alarming presentation, the videotapes of the 12 sessions showed impressive and rapid progress. While Mann was not a researcher, his ideas were stimulating and influential.

In contrast, the open-ended approach of long-term psychoanalysis runs the risk of stasis and regression. Freud (1937) struggled with this issue, as some of his treatments, which originally lasted for months, tended to drag on for years. What he did not consider was that therapy itself is somewhat addictive, and that goals are often set too high. This is why Alexander and French (1946) suggested replacing open-ended psychoanalysis with a series of shorter interventions with breaks in between to encourage patients to work on their own. This model could be modernized to offer brief therapy as the default condition, while leaving the door open for multiple courses of treatment. This is what we do in our BPD program (Paris, 2017).

Some may object that brief dynamic therapy is only a form of crisis intervention, as opposed to lengthier therapy that can lead to personality change. My reaction is – prove it! Without good evidence to justify seeing patients for years, we could well be satisfied with the evidence that real change can happen in a few months. This also means that effective treatment can become accessible to many more patients.

It is striking how many of the pioneers of brief therapy – Hans Strupp (Strupp and Binder, 1984), Lester Luborsky (Luborsky and Luborsky, 2006), David Malan (1980), Peter Sifneos (1979), Habib Davanloo (2001), and James Mann (1980) – were either trained psychoanalysts or psychodynamically oriented therapists. These clinicians were skeptical about the necessity of long-term treatment. In each of their models, patients were treated with somewhere between 10 and 20 well-focused sessions. They were pioneers in bringing the psychodynamic perspective to brief therapy, and in making its insights available to a much broader population.

A reduced role for long-term therapy

Some patients, even if they are in the minority, need more than brief psychotherapy. But we should be cautious about prescribing treatments that are not evidence-based. The patients who seem to need longer therapy are usually those with chronic problems such as severe personality disorders, addictions, or eating disorders. Yet in most clinical settings these cases will be in a minority. And given the potential that longer treatment tends to create waiting lists, long-term therapy should be regularly reviewed and monitored, to ensure that it is working.

Clinicians who practice brief therapy will be aware that patients who complete a course of treatment may often still have significant problems. To paraphrase one of Freud's witticisms, we can be satisfied to replace unnecessary misery with the normal suffering of human life.

However, even if they are not fully "cured", patients can still continue to apply the skills they learn on their own. Research shows that most patients continue to improve after termination of a successful treatment (Lambert,

2013). Also, when researchers have examined how fast patients improve in longer therapy, improvements still plateau out around six months. This is true even of therapies like DBT that target chronic suicidality (Stanley et al., 2007). Thus, even though it seems logical that long-term problems need long-term treatment, this is not necessarily the case.

Consider a classical study of the dose-effect relationship in psychotherapy conducted 30 years ago by Howard et al. (1986). Data were collected on more than 2,400 patients attending clinics over a 30-year period. Meta-analyses showed that by eight sessions approximately 50% of patients were measurably improved, and approximately 75% were improved by 26 sessions. Moreover, the 25% who did not improve did no better if seen for a full year. This study has never been repeated in the decades since it was published, and it still stands as the most impressive data on the question of how long therapy should usually last (Kopta, 2003). One might argue that the outcome measures were largely symptomatic, and that long-term therapy aims for personality change. But there is little evidence that lengthy treatment can achieve that goal.

What then should be the role for longer-term therapy? A more resource-intensive and expensive option could be insurable under certain circumstances, as is the case for many expensive treatments in medicine. For example, longer treatment could be reserved for patients who fail to benefit from shorter and more targeted interventions.

That sequence would be an example of a *stepped care* model, in which briefer therapy is offered to most patients, while longer treatments are reserved for those who fail the first step (Bower and Gilboody, 2005). This procedure helps ensure that long-term therapy is not offered routinely, and that it is prescribed for those who need it most. That population will almost certainly be dominated by patients with personality disorders (Paris, 2017).

While I agree with psychoanalysts (e.g., Leichsenring et al, 2015) who have suggested that complex psychopathology can *sometimes* require longer treatment, my own experience with treating patients with severe problems is that it is not necessarily required. My work with borderline personality disorder is based on reserving this option after trying briefer interventions that can be surprisingly efficacious (Paris, 2017). We have found that the majority of cases can be well managed with 12 individual and 12 group sessions (Laporte et al., 2018). Thus in our specialized clinics for BPD, longer-term therapy emphasizing rehabilitation is offered a backup option: either when brief therapy has been tried without success, or in patients with severe psychosocial dysfunction that leads to chronic unemployment and/or social isolation. Our experience over the last two decades shows that only 12% of cases treated briefly return for more therapy (Laporte et al., 2018). In BPD, which everyone agrees is a "complex" form of psychopathology, a recent systematic review concluded that a short course of therapy (around 14 sessions) is as effective as longer-term treatment (Links et al., 2017).

The problem with open-ended long-term therapy is that, as Alexander and French (1946) realized many decades ago, is that it has no end-point. Life is full of problems, so there is never a lack of issues to address. But psychological change will be limited by other factors, such as temperament and current life situations. Moreover, when treatment lasts for several years, how can one be sure that any observed improvements are the result of therapy, as opposed to maturation and/or changes in life circumstances?

In short, there is no such thing as being "completely" analyzed. This is a chimera that has never been supported by evidence. If clinicians wish to offer a longer therapy, they should be aware that this option is not evidence-based, and not promise their patients a "cure".

Research does not support seeing patients for years on end, always hoping for a breakthrough. That might be called the "Woody Allen syndrome". Wallerstein (2000), in a review of treatment at the Menninger Clinic, described patients who became what he called "lifers". I think that most of us will have seen patients who become addicted to psychotherapy. Or, as one of my colleagues once remarked, therapy can play the same role as a trip to the hairdresser.

Freud (1937) was the first to write about this issue. He started by treating patients briefly, but found many who were unwilling to leave therapy, or came back later with the same problems. But his conclusions about "interminable" analysis, that drives can be too powerful, was dubious. Instead, it makes more sense to view the goals of an ideal analysis as unreachable in principle. Instead, clinicians can aim for sufficient improvement that patients can continue the treatment on their own, becoming their own therapist. And if further problems come up later, therapy can be a "retread", with a similar time limit.

Another way to prevent drift and stasis in long-term therapy is to carry out regular re-evaluations. In our BPD clinics, patients are limited to about 18 months of therapy (both group and individual). But we meet with them every six months to review progress and to re-examine goals. While most patients are kept in the program after these reviews, this procedure allows us to discharge those who are not motivated towards progress. But when we advise patients to leave the program, we leave the door open to a further evaluation, when and if they feel more ready to get involved in treatment. These procedures, particularly the formal six-monthly re-evaluation, could also be applied in office practice.

Again, the problem that has troubled me throughout my career is that the demand for therapy greatly exceeds the supply of affordable treatment. It is worth keeping in mind that every time we treat patients over several years, we block places for other potential patients who need help, and might be managed more briefly. If there were a shortage of a flu vaccine, we would not ration it or raise the price, but would make sure it was available to everyone. The same principle should apply to psychotherapy. Psychodynamic therapy has something to offer to patients with a wide range of psychopathology, and it should not be reserved for the wealthy or the "worried well".

Some have argued that critiques of open-ended therapy fail to validate the suffering of people who are willing to undergo psychoanalysis. Doidge et al. (2002) conducted a survey showing that most patients in analysis meet formal criteria for diagnoses listed in the DSM manual. But this may only prove that DSM-5 is over-inclusive, and that it pathologizes normal variations (Frances, 2013). Of course, people who seek therapy are troubled and unhappy. But that does not mean that every treatment needs to be lengthy and make personality change its goal. I am not saying that one should *never* offer patients long-term therapy. But if we do so, we need to monitor the process closely. And as proposed long ago by Alexander and French (1946), therapy can be *intermittent* rather than continuous. If clinicians are not blinded by a belief in perfection, we can see patients in multiple courses of treatment at different stages of their development.

I once asked my own psychoanalyst, a local leader in his profession, for his views on this issue. He suggested that formal, long-term therapy should be reserved for training purposes, and that most patients would benefit from more streamlined treatment. Given the strong evidence for briefer therapy, and the much weaker evidence for longer therapy, this position is now justified by empirical data.

One might ask whether a more restricted view of long-term therapy would actually make brief therapy more available. I think it would, but I cannot cite evidence to prove my impression. What I can say is in my years of experience with hospital and community clinics, therapists who are not made accountable, and are allowed to see patients for as long as they think necessary, conduct a practice in which long-standing patients are followed so that new patients cannot enter treatment. Unless there are rules supporting accountability, out-patient clinics get blocked. And even in private practice, where patients are paying for a service and might therefore be considered to have the right to stay if they wish, the situation does not reflect evidence-based practice, and does not make a contribution to meeting population needs.

Models of brief psychodynamic therapy

In the 1970s, several psychoanalysts developed models of brief therapy based on dynamic principles. David Malan (1980), whose approach to therapy derived from the British school of object relations, suggested that brief therapy can benefit from the use of transference interpretations. However, these conclusions have not been supported by later research. Another figure in the same generation was the American analyst Peter Sifneos (1979), but his focus on Oedipal issues would seem out of date today (and has not been validated by research). And as much as I admired the ideas of James Mann (1980), there is no evidence that his approach is any better than alternative methods.

Habib Davanloo (2001), who worked for many years in my department, was not formally trained in psychoanalysis, but was a charismatic therapist who convinced others through strongly held convictions. His method of brief therapy was once written up in the *New York Times* (Sobel, 1982), underlining that Davanloo, unlike almost anyone else at the time, made videotapes of his therapy sessions, rather than confining himself to case reports that can be far from the raw data of practice.

Yet none of these investigators were trained researchers, and their methodology would not meet current standards. And given the strong evidence that brief therapies do not differ from each other in outcome (Wampold, 2001), it is likely that the technical interventions described by pioneers in the field were less crucial than they thought. The studies that have shown the effectiveness of brief psychodynamic therapy (Shapiro et al., 2003; Leichsenring et al., 2015; Steinert et al., 2017) have not followed particular model or system. Luborsky (2006), a pioneer in psychotherapy research, and who conducted more rigorous research on brief therapy, was interested in a wide variety of psychodynamic themes, but the thrust of his ideas was to focus on relational issues.

Today, research on the process and outcome of brief dynamic therapy remains active, conducted mainly by research groups in the UK, the US, and Germany. But research need not be associated with any specific acronym or charismatic clinician. That is all to the good. The field is maturing beyond an initial stage of adherence to various founders, backed up only by theory and case reports. Practitioners should be reading journals that publish research articles with high clinical relevance. Brief psychodynamic therapy, now firmly evidence-based, has become part of mainstream clinical psychology. But successful clinical work can be boosted by an eclecticism that is open to new ideas from any source.

Conclusion

Classical psychoanalysis has not made a contribution to population needs for psychotherapy. It is long, expensive, and not well based in evidence. Taking a public-health approach, we need to adapt the treatment and use its insights in a different way, by making it shorter, less expensive, and more evidence-based. The best option for most patients is brief therapy lasting three to six months, with the door left open for later re-assessment. Long-term therapy should no longer be the first recommendation, but a backup option with a different time limit and with specific goals.

References

Abbass, A., Town, J., Driessen, E.: Intensive short-term dynamic psychotherapy: A systematic review and meta-analysis of outcome research. *Harvard Review of Psychiatry* 2012, 20: 97–108.

Alexander, F., French, T.: *Psychoanalytic Therapy*. New York, Ronald Press, 1946.

Bower, P., Gilboody, S.: Stepped care in psychological therapies: Access, effectiveness and efficiency. *British Journal of Psychiatry* 2005, 186: 11–17.

Chamberlin, J.: Survey says: More Americans are seeking mental health treatment. *Monitor on Psychology* July/August 2004, 17–20.

Clark, D.M.: Realizing the mass public benefit of Evidence-Based Psychological Therapies: The IAPT program. *Annual Review of Clinical Psychology* 2018, 14: 159–183.

Cuijpers, P., Van Straten, A., Andersson, G., van Oppen, P.: Psychotherapy for depression in adults: A meta-analysis of comparative outcome studies. *Journal of Consulting and Clinical Psychology* 2008, 76: 909–922.

Davanloo, J.: *Intensive Short-Term Dynamic Psychotherapy*. New York, Springer, 2001.

Doidge, N., Simon, B., Brauer, L., Grant, D.C., First, M., Brunshaw, J., Lancee, W.J., Stevens, A., Oldham, J.M., Mosher, P.: Psychoanalytic patients in the U.S., Canada,

and Australia: I. DSM-III-R disorders, indications, previous treatment, medications, and length of treatment. *Journal of the American Psychoanalytic Association* 2002, 50: 575–614.
Eagle, M.: *From Classical to Contemporary Psychoanalysis: A Critique and Integration.* New York, Routledge, 2011.
Frances, A.: *Saving Normal.* New York, Harper Collins, 2013.
Freud, S.: Analysis terminable and interminable. *International Journal of Psychoanalysis* 1937, 18: 373–385.
Gerber, A.J., Kocsis, J.H., Milrod, B.L., Roose, S.P., Barber, J.P., Thase, M.E., Perkins, P., Leon, A.C.: A quality-based review of randomized controlled trials of psychodynamic psychotherapy. *American Journal of Psychiatry* 2011, 168: 19–28.
Goldbeck-Wood, S.: The future of psychotherapy in the NHS. *BMJ* 2004, 329: 245.
Han, B., Hedden, S.L., Lipari, R., Copello, E., Kroutil, L.A.: Receipt of services for behavioral health problems. *Substance Abuse and Mental Health Services Administration,* 2015. www.samhsa.gov/data/sites/default/files/NSDUH-DR-FRR3-2014/NSDUH-DR-FRR3-2014/NSDUH-DR-FRR3-2014.htm.
Hemmings, A.: A systematic review of the effectiveness of brief psychological therapies in primary health care. *Families, Systems, & Health* 2000, 18: 279–313.
Howard, K.I., Kopta, S.M., Krause, M.S., Orlinsky, D.E.: The dose-effect relationship to psychotherapy. *American Psychologist* 1986, 41: 159–164.
Johnson, L.D.: Psychotherapy in the age of accountability. *Journal of Nervous and Mental Diseases* 1996, 184: 259–265.
Kessler, R.C., Chiu, W.T., Demler, O., Merikangas, K.R., Walters, E.E.: Prevalence, severity, and comorbidity of 12-month DSM-IV disorders in the National Comorbidity Survey replication. *Archives of General Psychiatry* 2005, 62: 617–627.
Kopta, S.M.: The dose-effect relationship in psychotherapy: A defining achievement for Dr. Kenneth Howard. *Journal of Clinical Psychology* 2003, 59: 727–733.
Lambert, M.: *Handbook of Psychotherapy and Behavior Change.* New York, Wiley, 2013.
Laporte, L., Paris, J., Zelkowitz, P., Cardin, J.F.: Clinical outcomes of Stepped Care for the treatment of borderline personality disorder. *Personality and Mental Health,* 12: 252–264, 2018.
Lazar, S.G.: The cost-effectiveness of psychotherapy for the major psychiatric diagnoses. *Psychodynamic Psychiatry* 2014, 42: 423–457.
Leichensring, F., Luyten, P., Hilsenroth, M.J., Abbass, A., Barber, J.P., Keefe, J.R., Leweke, F., Rabung, S., Steinert, C.: Psychodynamic therapy meets evidence-based medicine: A systematic review using updated criteria. *Lancet Psychiatry* 2015, 2: 648–660.
Leichsenring, F., Rabung, S.: Effectiveness of long-term psychodynamic psychotherapy: A meta-analysis. *JAMA* 2008, 300: 1551–1565.
Levenson, H., Davidovitz, D.: Brief therapy prevalence and training: A national survey of psychologists. *Psychotherapy* 2000, 37: 335–340.
Links, P.S., Shah, R., Eynan, R.: Psychotherapy for borderline personality disorder: Progress and remaining challenges. *Current Psychiatry Reports* 2017, 19: 16.
Luborsky, L., Luborsky, E.: *Research and Psychotherapy: The Vital Link.* Lanham, MD, Jason Aronson, 2006.
Malan, D.: *A Study of Brief Psychotherapy.* London, Springer, 1980.
Mann, J.: *Time-Limited Psychotherapy.* Cambridge, MA, Harvard University Press, 1980.
McHugh, R.K., Whitton, S.W., Peckham, A.F., Welge, J.A., Otto, M.W.: Patient preference for psychological vs. pharmacological treatment of psychiatric disorders: A meta-analytic review. *Journal of Clinical Psychiatry* 2013, 74: 595–602.

Olfson, M., Marcus, S.C.: National trends in outpatient psychotherapy. *American Journal of Psychiatry* 2010, 167: 1456–1463.

Olfson, M., Marcus, S.M., Druss, B., Pincus, H.A.: National trends in the use of outpatient psychotherapy. *American Journal of Psychiatry* 2002, 159: 1914–1920.

Paris, J.: *Psychotherapy in an Age of Neuroscience*. New York, Oxford University Press, 2016.

Paris, J.: *Stepped Care for Borderline Personality Disorder*. New York, Academic Press, 2017.

Seligman, M.E.P.: The effectiveness of psychotherapy: The consumer reports study. *American Psychologist* 1995, 50: 965–974.

Shapiro, D.A., Barkham, M., Hardy, G.E., Rees, A., Reynolds, S., Startup, M.: Time is of the essence: A selective review of the fall and rise of brief therapy research. *Psychology and Psychotherapy* 2003, 76: 211–235.

Sifneos, P.: *Short-Term Dynamic Psychotherapy: Evaluation and Technique*. New York, Springer, 1979.

Smit, Y., Huibers, J., Ioannidis, J., van Dyck, R., van Tilburg, W., Arntz, A.: The effectiveness of long-term psychoanalytic psychotherapy: A meta-analysis of randomized controlled trials. *Clinical Psychology Review* 2012, 32: 81–92.

Sobel, D.: A new and controversial short-term psychotherapy. *New York Times*, November 21, 1982.

Stanley, B., Brodsky, B., Nelson, J., Dulit, R.: Brief dialectical behavior therapy for suicidality and self-injurious behaviors. *Archives of Suicide Research* 2007, 11: 337–341.

Steinert, C, Munder, T, Rabung, S, Hoyer, J, Leichsenring, F (2017): Psychodynamic Therapy: As efficacious as other empirically supported treatments? A meta-analysis testing equivalence of outcomes *Am J Psychiatry* 174: 943–953.

Strupp, H., Binder, J.: *Psychotherapy in a New Key: A Guide to Time-Limited Dynamic Psychotherapy*. New York, Basic Books, 1984.

Substance Abuse and Mental Health Administration: *More Americans Continue to Receive Mental Health Services, But Substance Use Treatment Levels Remain Low*, 2015. www.samhsa.gov/data/sites/default/files/NSDUH-DR-FRR3-2014/NSDUH-DR-FRR3-2014/NSDUH-DR-FRR3-2014.htm, accessed March 7, 2018.

Summers, R.F., Barber, J.: *Psychodynamic Therapy: A Guide to Evidence-Based Practice*. New York, Guilford Press, 2012.

Wallerstein, R.: *42 Lives in Treatment*. New York, Other Press, 2000.

Wampold, B.E.: *The Great Psychotherapy Debate: Models, Methods, and Findings*. Mahwah, NJ, Erlbaum Associates, 2001.

Part II

The boundaries of psychoanalysis

Chapter 6

Psychoanalysis and neuroscience

Neuroscience and psychopathology

The mind is a product of the brain, and neuroscience has developed powerful tools to measure brain activity. Advances in technology have made it possible to measure correlates of thoughts and emotions through imaging. The beautiful pictures (albeit with artificial colors) produced by functional magnetic resonance imaging (fMRI) seem to support the assumption that the mind can be understood by observing activity in various brain regions.

Neuroscience has become a cutting edge of research in psychology. Brain imaging is increasingly being used to validate broader scientific constructs. Measure of brain functioning, either as the foundation of empirical research, or as an add-on to measures of mental phenomena, are being applied to widen the scope of research on the mind.

These developments have offered a new opening for theorists who wish to root psychoanalysis in research. Thus, if psychological data on a mental level fail to confirm some psychoanalytic tenets, is there a way to support Freud's theories by correlating them with neurobiological findings?

Neuroscience, particularly fMRI, is being used to support the current view that mental processes can be accounted for by neural connections. This research program is highly influential in research on psychopathology. The National Institute of Mental Health requires applicants for grants to link hypotheses to their neuroscience-based model. The Research Domain Criteria (RDoC) are a set of descriptors that classify mental disorders on the basis of changes in neuroconnectivity, and which aim to become a new way to classify and understand psychopathology (Cuthbert and Insel, 2013). Many neuroscientists are excited about this approach, which aims eventually to replace the biologically imprecise categories listed in the Diagnostic and Statistical Manual, 5th edition (DSM-5; American Psychiatric Association, 2013).

Yet there is a big problem with RDoC. The current level of knowledge in neuroscience is insufficiently developed to support the project (Paris and Kirmayer, 2016). We do not know enough about the brain to explain the mind, or about the mind to know how to study the brain. This proposal is, in the well-known phrase, "a bridge too far". In spite of great progress over the last 20 years, neuroscience is still in its infancy. That is inevitable, given the task of explaining thought, emotion, and behavior through the activity and connections of nearly 100 billion neurons.

Another problem is that RDoC implicitly devalues psychosocial research, not to speak of psychotherapy. Yet it is now widely recognized that talking therapy can change the brain, as research has documented (Goldapple et al., 2004). In this way, psychotherapy is as potent a modifier of neural connections as any drug. However, RDoC's agenda seems to require psychological research to be validated on a cellular level.

A belief in *reductionism* (i.e., accounting for phenomena by examining processes at a more fundamental level), threatens to turn psychology into neuroscience, and has driven many psychiatrists to treat psychological problems almost exclusively with medication (Paris, 2017). Similar trends have affected academic psychology, as the most prestigious psychology departments provide major financial support to build laboratories for neuroscience research. Clinical psychologists, although they do not prescribe medication, can also be influenced by this climate of opinion, and sometimes encourage their patients to see physicians to be put on antidepressants. Finally, patients are influenced by the media, which love a good story better than the uncertainties of real science. The media like to promulgate the idea that brain imaging can explain the mind.

The prestige of neuroscience has led to many new fields of inquiry in the academic world. Some, such as neuropsychology and neuropsychiatry, have long histories. Others are new: neuro-ethics, neuro-economics, neuro-engineering, neuro-criminology, and neuro-criticism. Thus, the prefix "neuro" has become a way of validating entire lines of research and scholarship (Satel and Lilienfeld, 2013). This trend has now spread to psychoanalysis.

The birth of neuropsychoanalysis

A group of psychoanalysts, led by the South African neuropsychologist Mark Solms, founded a movement that aims to use neuroscience to support Freud's theories of the mind (Solms and Turnbull, 2002; Panksepp and Solms, 2012). The idea is to map brain activity, using fMRI to identify those areas that "light up" in correlation with various states of mind, most particularly with the constructs of classical psychoanalysis.

The problem is that, instead of building up a model of the mind from our current knowledge of neuroscience, the proponents of neuropsychoanalysis begin with a pre-existing hundred-year-old model which they aimed to validate. But there is a huge gap between psychoanalytical theories of the mind and what can be observed in brain scans.

Moreover, while fMRI is a powerful technology, it has major limitations. It should be kept in mind that the pictures of brain regions we see in scientific journals (and in the media) are averages drawn from many subjects, and represent the activity of thousands of neurons that may or may not have a common function. This is why neuroscience, like so many other scientific domains, faces a "replication crisis", in which findings are reported, but all too often contradicted. As one neuroscientist has commented (Raz, 2012, p. 268):

> fMRI studies frequently produce billions of data points – most of them sheer noise – wherein one can find coincidental patterns. Whirl those tea leaves around often enough and recognizable impressions will appear at the bottom of your cup. In addition, many fMRI studies dip into the same data twice: first to pick out which parts of the brain are responding; and second to measure the response strength. This practice is statistically problematic and results in findings that appear stronger than they actually are.

I have lived long enough to see my own discipline of psychiatry dominated by two strongly held but opposing ideas: the first being psychoanalysis, and the second being neuroscience. In today's intellectual climate, neuroscience is the clear winner, and psychological constructs may only be taken seriously if they have measurable neural correlates. This explains why, to address the decline in the prestige of psychoanalysis, an attempt has been made to root its model in neurobiological research.

Unfortunately, the starting point is not modern psychoanalysis, which is moving closer to mainstream psychology, but Freud's original model (Solms and Turnbull, 2002). The claim that newer methods of studying the brain can validate these ideas, which have not previously been found to be consistent with modern neuroscience, is very doubtful.

The founder of this movement, Mark Solms, began his career by studying brain-damaged patients. This work may have convinced him that the mind has precise equivalents in the brain. Solms founded a society holding annual conferences devoted to neuropsychoanalysis, as well as a dedicated scientific journal of the same name. His supporters in this venture have included the famous neurologist Oliver Sacks, who wrote a preface to one of Solms' books. (In an autobiography, Sacks [2015] described his own experiences as a patient in psychoanalysis over many decades, suggesting that he was far from a disinterested observer.)

Solms attracted further attention by publishing an article in *Scientific American* entitled "Freud Returns" (Solms, 2006). Arguing that most of the key ideas behind psychoanalysis can be validated by neuroscience research, the titles of several sections of the article indicate the ground he covered: "unconscious motivation", "repression vindicated", "pleasure principle", "animal within", and "dreams have meaning".

First and foremost, Solms claims that cognitive neuroscience confirms the Freudian unconscious. He gave the example of confabulations that arise from a lesion in the cingulate gyrus of the cerebral cortex, goes on to claim that repression is supported by research studies, and concludes that the dopamine system corresponds to Freud's pleasure principle. Solms continues by referencing Paul MacLean's (1990) theory of a triune brain, with layers that range from the most primitive (the reptilian brain) to the most advanced (the human brain), claiming that they correspond to the id, ego, and superego. Actually, MacLean's theory, while often quoted, has been questioned, given that a well-developed cerebral cortex can be found in most non-mammalian species (Striedter, 2005). Finally, Solms argued that Freud's theory of dreams as wish fulfillments is supported by neuroscientific research.

Unfortunately, *Scientific American* did not publish commentaries discussing the many problems associated with these dazzling leaps of theory. But recognizing how controversial his claims were, Solms included a nod to critics, writing (2006, p. 88):

> For older neuroscientists, resistance to the return of psychoanalytical ideas comes from the specter of the seemingly indestructible edifice of Freudian theory in the early years of their careers. They cannot acknowledge even partial confirmation of Freud's fundamental insights; they demand a complete purge. In the words of J. Alan

> Hobson, a renowned sleep researcher and Harvard Medical School psychiatrist, the renewed interest in Freud is little more than unhelpful "retrofitting" of modern data into an antiquated theoretical framework. But as Panksepp said in a 2002 interview with *Newsweek* magazine, for neuroscientists who are enthusiastic about the reconciliation of neurology and psychiatry, "it is not a matter of proving Freud right or wrong, but of finishing the job".

In the end, most of Solms' claims are either dubious or based on "cherry-picking" the neuroscience literature. The correspondences between Freudian theory and fMRI data are superficial, and hardly support the complex but shaky edifice of classical psychoanalytic theory.

Let us focus on the key idea of neuropsychoanalysis, that mechanisms governing the unconscious mind can be observed through neuroimaging. It has long been known that when people make decisions, changes in the brain can be observed even before these thoughts enter consciousness (Libet, 1985). But while this data supports the existence of an unconscious mind, it says nothing about its *content*. Correlations between analytic constructs and brain regions can be interpreted in many ways. Thus claims that a marriage of psychoanalysis and neuroscience is on the horizon are at best premature. The research literature remains thin, and it does not put much meat on these bones.

We can also consider the relation of neuroscience to dreams. Solms has suggested that Freud's ideas about dreams are consistent with current neuroscience, and with research based on REM activity. This attempt to rescue the older theory has met with opposition from dream researchers, who consider Freud's clinical speculations to be incompatible with empirical data (Hobson, 2015; Domhoff, 2004).

Neuroscientists have paid scant attention to the claims of neuropsychoanalysis, and tend to see links to psychology as lying in cognitive science. The proposal to establish a new discipline also met with a mixed reception from traditional psychoanalysts, many of whom do not want to dilute Freud's wine with neuroscientific water (Blass and Carmeli, 2007).

In summary, neuropsychoanalysis suffers from being used to support long-standing models, without attempting to find something new, or to develop an integration based on the perspectives of current psychological research. Much of the support for the idea has come from outside observers. There are hardly any published papers on the subject outside psychoanalytic journals. The main exception was the late Jan Panskeep, a Dutch neuroscientist, who was one of Solm's co-authors.

Eric Kandel, a psychiatrist and neuroscience researcher, became influential after he won a Nobel Prize for the study of the neurochemistry of memory. Kandel (1998) has taken a sympathetic view of the use of biological methods to study psychoanalytic theory. In his autobiography, Kandel (2007) explains that he had wanted to be an analyst before choosing neuroscience. Yet since he became a full-time researcher and gave up the practice of psychiatry, Kandel may be caught in a time warp. While he is an expert on the chemistry of memory in the sea slug, he seems unaware that psychoanalysis is not the only form of psychotherapy, and that it has changed over time to avoid being overtaken by competitors.

The science journalist Casey Schwartz has published an admiring book on neuropsychoanalysis (Schwartz, 2015), well reviewed in the *New York Times*. A section of her book excerpted in the *New York Times Magazine* (June 24, 2015), was provocatively titled: "Tell it about your mother: can brain scanning save Freudian psychoanalysis?"

In these publications, Schwartz quotes the work of two psychoanalyst-researchers, Andrew Gerber, and Bradley Peterson at UCLA, who state they are able to visualize the process of transference in the brain (Gerber and Peterson, 2006; Gerber et al., 2015). These claims should raise eyebrows, as psychotherapy researchers have not found this construct easy to measure, and there have been only a limited number of empirical studies of transference phenomena (Luborsky and Crits-Christoph, 1998; Piper, 1991). The studies that impressed Schwartz used a dubious method of assessment in which psychoanalysts fill out questionnaires about their patients. It is well known in research that therapists are not the best people to ask about what is going in sessions (Norcross, 2011). Schwartz goes on to describe interviews with other leading figures who support these views: Erich Kandel, Otto Kernberg, and Glen Gabbard. Unfortunately, Schwartz's "gee whiz" description is sorely lacking in tough-minded assessments of this "new science".

To understand why neuropsychoanalysis is not mainstream science, we need to take a more critical look at its assumptions and conclusions. First and foremost, it begins with the assumption that Freud was right about almost everything, and the role of research is to prove that he was. No serious attempt is made to say what parts of the theory should be kept, and what should be modified or discarded.

Second, there is very little data to support its sweeping claims. Most of the articles on the subject present theoretical generalizations and hopeful claims about the future.

Third, the methods used to measure psychoanalytic concepts are embarrassingly primitive. Asking psychoanalysts to rate what patients tell them is even more invalid that asking patients what they thought was accomplished.

Fourth, the idea of localizing mental functions in specific brain regions is itself problematic. Circuitry governing thought, emotions, and behavior is widely distributed in the brain (Andreasen, 2001; Kagan, 2017). While some mental functions can be localized, most involve the coordinated activity of many brain regions.

In summary, brain scans cannot be used to support psychoanalytic theory. Even in general psychiatry, imaging tells you little more than you can observe by spending time talking with a patient. To support psychoanalysis with research, we need to study the mind on a mental level, conducting systematic research on its theories, and on the efficacy of its method in practice. We are decades away from any application of neuroscience that could short-circuit this project. Neuropsychoanalysis amounts to a game of "see, Freud was right all along – I told you so, and you see it on a brain scan". This is not an answer to a very complex problem.

Neuroplasticity

Another proposal for the use of neuroscience to support psychoanalysis depends on the concept of *neuroplasticity*. This is the principle that the brain can modify its circuits in adult life – and that psychotherapy can change this circuitry. It has been shown that psychotherapeutic interventions produce changes that can be observed using imaging methods (e.g., Goldapple et al., 2004). Thus, there can be little doubt that psychotherapy *does* change the brain. (If it didn't, it is hard to see how it could ever work.)

It used to be thought that neurons in the brain cannot be replaced and stop growing in the adult years. But recent research, summarized by Costandi (2016), shows that neurogenesis does occur in some brain regions (particularly the hippocampus), and that connections between neurons continue to change throughout the life cycle. Moreover, even if neurons are not replaced, they can form new connections. It is also known that when brain regions are damaged, other regions can, at least to some extent, take over their functions. In this way, research has confirmed theories concerning the formation of neural networks developed many decades ago by the Canadian psychologist Donald Hebb (1949), i.e., that "neurons that fire together wire together".

Thus, the evidence for neuroplasticity is strong, and generally supports the idea that psychological (or biological) interventions can, at least to some extent, rewire the brain. However, it is not established whether these effects are strong enough to reverse severe and chronic mental illnesses. Claims that they can accomplish such miracles go well beyond the evidence.

In a popular book, the Canadian psychoanalyst Norman Doidge (2007) reviewed this literature, reaching the hopeful conclusion that psychotherapy can dramatically change the brain. I found the book stimulating, but was less impressed with a chapter arguing that the practice of psychoanalysis is specifically supported by these observations.

After the first volume became a best-seller, Doidge (2015) wrote a second book that went much further. Doidge claimed that mental exercises can reverse the course of severe neurological and psychiatric problems, including chronic pain, stroke, multiple sclerosis, Parkinson's disease, and autism. Doidge's claim was that each of these conditions can be treated with procedures using mental imagery and cognitive control. Thus, stroke would be treated with "functional integration lessons", Parkinson's disease with "conscious walking", multiple sclerosis with electrical stimulation of the tongue, and autistic spectrum disorder with music and voices of changing frequencies.

Unfortunately, almost all of Doidge's ideas were based on anecdotes rather than solid research, failing to meet any of the standards of scientific research. For this reason, they had little impact in medicine or neuroscience. They have not been accepted for publication in scientific journals, but were described in a book written for a popular audience.

The only comment I could find by an expert was from the British geriatrician and researcher Raymond Tallis (2015), who wrote a critical review of the book in the Wall Street Journal. As he comments:

> Dr. Doidge's pen portraits of patients facing neurological adversity with courage and determination, and of their charismatic healers, are disarming. Yet the reliance on anecdotes and testimonials, without much clinically and scientifically relevant detail, is exasperating. . . . It seemed

> reasonable to conclude that, while using what we currently know of neuroplasticity may deliver modest therapeutic advances, we need to learn much more about the brain before we can hope to regularly achieve the results that Dr. Doidge reports.

Even so, Doidge's ideas were headlined on the Canadian Broadcasting Company's television program "The Nature of Things". Hosted by the geneticist David Suzuki, this series has been a leading venue for popularizing science in Canada. But to hear Suzuki say on TV that Doidge has created a revolution in neurology was dispiriting. (Evidently Suzuki does not do his own script writing, and texts are prepared by his staff.) At one point in the documentary, Doidge actually advises a skeptic to "suspend disbelief". One has to be a true believer oneself to take such an unscientific view of the world.

This story shows why evidence-based medicine needs to be the basis of modern psychiatry. Although the public, as well as medical journalists, can be impressed with anecdotes, physicians with a scientific training are only satisfied with hard evidence. Unfortunately, the media love a good story better than facts. This is how books, however marked by misinformation, sometimes become best-sellers. They create false hopes, which, however unrealistic, have a certain appeal to patients and families. Unfortunately, these speculations are likely to lead disillusionment.

A better way: cognitive neuroscience and psychoanalysis

Cognitive science is a relatively new branch of psychological research developed about 40 years ago. (The related term, *cognitive neuroscience*, is a discipline that emphasizes the use of fMRI to study mental processes.)

These disciplines concern the scientific study of how people think. Several researchers and theoreticians, noting that Freud's theory of the mind is not compatible with contemporary psychological research, have proposed that psychoanalysis could benefit from establishing links with these research programs (Colby and Stoller, 1988). Wilma Bucci (1998) was a psychoanalyst who explored this idea in detail, developing what she called "multiple code theory", i.e., emphasized emotional information processing and the development of emotion schemas as central in an individual's representation of the world. Bucci's model is clearly incompatible with classical theory, as it sees the function of the mind not as drive reduction, but information processing. These ideas are consistent with mainstream neuroscience.

Fonagy and Target (2007) noted that cognitive science is more consistent with attachment theory than with classical psychoanalysis. It is consistent with a tendency to replace a theory of drives with a focus on interpersonal relationships and emotional responses. Similarly, the Italian analyst-researcher Antonio Imbasciati (2003) has argued that cognitive science is not compatible with drive theory, but might be reconciled with object relations theories. (These developments were discussed in Chapter 4.)

Establishing links to cognitive science could be useful. Westen (1998) noted several areas of overlap with psychoanalysis, such the nature of mental representations, the interaction of cognition and affect, and the mechanisms by which the mind make compromises when they conflict. Ruby (2013) suggested that this interface could be used to go beyond observable data to study the role of meaning in mental activity – an issue that tends to be absent from the cognitive approach. At the present time, these ideas are very general and unlikely to contribute to the development of theory and practice. The best one can say is that it is better to use cognitive science as a starting point, rather than beginning with the outdated ideas of Freud in the hopes of validating them.

Conclusions

Neuroscience is a discipline that is still very young. It is not ready to explain the complex workings of the human mind or the treatment of mental illness. Many of its ideas are suggestive and stimulating. For example, the discovery of "mirror neurons" in which the brain tracks the motivations and emotions of others, has been thought relevant to psychoanalysis (Gallese et al., 2007). However other neuroscientists have found the concept over-hyped and much more complex than originally thought (Hickock, 2014).

It is possible to envisage a time when the progress of patients in treatment will be monitored by imaging technology. But even if that were to happen, one cannot reduce the complexity of the mind to brain circuitry. A better start would be to establish links with cognitive science, which, like psychoanalysis and academic psychology, studies the mind on a mental level. Some psychoanalysts, such as Gabbard (2000), have promoted a neurobiologically informed perspective on psychotherapy. However, our knowledge of neuroscience is still too primitive to allow any useful clinical applications.

References

American Psychiatric Association: *Diagnostic and Statistical Manual of Mental Disorders*, 5th edition. Washington, DC, American Psychiatric Publishing, 2013.

Andreasen, N.C.: *Brave New Brain: Conquering Mental Illness in the Era of the Genome*. New York, Oxford University Press, 2001.

Blass, R.B., Carmeli, Z.: The case against neuropsychoanalysis: On fallacies underlying psychoanalysis' latest scientific trend and its negative impact on psychoanalytic discourse. *International Journal of Psychoanalysis* 2007, 88: 19–40.

Bucci, W.: *Psychoanalysis and Cognitive Science: A Multiple Code Theory*. New York, Guilford Press, 1988.

Colby, K.M., Stoller, R.: *Cognitive Science and Psychoanalysis*. New York, Laurence Erlbaum, 1988.

Costandi, M.: *Neuroplasticity*. Cambridge, MA, MIT Press, 2016.

Cuthbert, B.N., Insel, T.R.: Toward the future of psychiatric diagnosis: The seven pillars of RDoC. *BMC Medicine* 2013, 11: 126.

Doidge, N.: *The Brain That Changes Itself*. New York, Penguin, 2007.

Doidge, N.: *The Brain's Way of Healing*. New York, Penguin, 2015.

Domhoff, G.W.: Why did empirical dream researchers reject Freud? A critique of historical claims by Mark Solms. *Dreaming* 2004, 14: 3–17.

Fonagy, P., Target, M.: The rooting of the mind in the body: New links between attachment theory and psychoanalytic thought. *Journal of the American Psychoanalytic Association* 2007, 55: 411–456.

Gabbard, G.O.: A neurobiologically informed perspective on psychotherapy. *British Journal of Psychiatry* 2000, 177: 117–122.

Gallese, V., Eagle, M., Mignone, P.: Intentional attunement: Mirror neurons and the neural underpinnings of interpersonal relations. *Journal of the American Psychoanalytic Association* 2007, 55: 131–175.

Gerber, A.J., Peterson, B.: Measuring transference phenomena with fMRI. *Journal of the American Psychoanalytic Association* 2006, 54: 1319–1325.

Gerber, A.J., Vinder, J., Roffman, J.: Neuroscience and psychoanalysis. In P. Luyten, L.C. Mayes, P. Fonagy, M. Target, S.J. Blatt, eds.: *Handbook of Psychodynamic Approaches to Psychopathology*. New York, Guilford Press, 2015, pp. 65–86.

Goldapple, K., Segal, Z., Garson, C., Kennedy, S.D., Mayberg, L.: Modulation of cortical-limbic pathways in major depression: Treatment-specific effects of cognitive behavior therapy. *Archives of General Psychiatry* 2004, 61: 34–41.

Hebb, D.O.: *The Organization of Behavior*. New York, Wiley, 1949.

Hickock, G.: *The Myth of Mirror Neurons: The Real Neuroscience of Communication and Cognition*. New York, Norton, 2014.

Hobson, J.A.: *Psychodynamic Neurology: Dreams, Consciousness, and Virtual Reality*. New York, Taylor & Francis, 2015.

Imbasciati, A.: Cognitive sciences and psychoanalysis: A possible convergence. *Journal of the American Academy of Psychoanalysis and Dynamic Psychiatry* 2003, 31: 627–646.

Kagan, J.: *Five Constraints on Predicting Behavior*. Cambridge, MA, MIT Press, 2017.
Kandel, E.R.: A new intellectual framework for psychiatry. *American Journal of Psychiatry* 1998, 155: 457–469.
Kandel, E.R.: *In Search of Memory: The Emergence of a New Science of Mind*. New York, W. W. Norton, 2007.
Libet, B.: Unconscious cerebral initiative and the role of conscious will in voluntary action. *Behavioral and Brain Sciences* 1985, 8: 529–566.
Luborsky, L., Crits-Christoph, P.: *Understanding Transference: The Core Conflictual Relationship Theme Method*, 2nd edition. Washington, DC, American Psychological Association, 1998.
MacLean, P.D.: *The Triune Brain in Evolution: Role in Paleocerebral Functions*. New York, Plenum Press, 1990.
Norcross, J.C., ed.: *Psychotherapy Relationships That Work: Evidence-Based Responsiveness*, 2nd edition. New York, Oxford University Press, 2011.
Panksepp, J., Solms, M.: What is neuropsychoanalysis? Clinically relevant studies of the minded brain. *Trends in Cognitive Science* 2012, 16: 6–8.
Paris, J.: *Psychotherapy in an Age of Neuroscience*. New York, Oxford University Press, 2017.
Paris, J., Kirmayer, L.J.: The NIMH research domain criteria: A bridge too far. *Journal of Nervous and Mental Disease* 2016, 204: 26–32.
Piper, W.E., Azim, H., Joyce, A.S.: Transference interpretations, therapeutic alliance, and outcome in short-term individual psychotherapy. *Archives of General Psychiatry* 1991, 48: 946–953.
Raz, A.: From neuroimaging to tea leaves in the bottom of a cup. In S. Choudhury, J. Slaby, eds.: *Critical Neuroscience*. New York, Wiley-Blackwell, 2012, pp. 265–270.
Ruby, P.: What would be the benefits of a collaboration between psychoanalysis and cognitive neuroscience? The opinion of a neuroscientist. *Frontiers in Human Neurosocience* 2013, 7: 475–485.
Sacks, O.: *On the Move*. London, Picador, 2015.
Satel, S., Lilienfeld, S.: *Brainwashed: The Seductive Appeal of Mindless Neuroscience*. New York, Basic Books, 2013.
Schwartz, C.: *In the Mind Fields: Exploring the New Science of Neuropsychoanalysis*. New York, Pantheon Books, 2015.
Solms, M.: Freud returns. *Scientific American*, April 2006, 17: 83–89.
Solms, M., Turnbull, O.: *The Brain and the Inner World: An Introduction to the Neuroscience of Subjective Experience*. London/New York, Other/Karnak, 2002.
Striedter, G.F.: *Principles of Brain Evolution*. New York, Oxford University Press, 2005.
Tallis, R.: Brainstorms brewing. *The Wall Street Journal*, February 27, 2015.
Westen, D.: The scientific legacy of Sigmund Freud: Toward a psychodynamically informed psychological science. *Psychological Bulletin* 1998, 124: 333–371.

Chapter 7

Nature, nurture, and psychoanalysis

The nature-nurture problem

The *nature-nurture problem* describes a long-standing debate between the belief that human nature is relatively fixed by biology, vs. the belief that the environment is the main force driving human development. This has long been a contentious issue in psychology and psychiatry.

The nature-nurture problem has also been a key issue in defining the relationship of psychoanalysis to other domains of research. While Freud (1930) acknowledged a role for "constitution" in development, and his drive theory focused on biological givens, he was vague about the details. But modern psychoanalytic theories, such as attachment theory and relational psychoanalysis, tend to give a crucial role to life experience and tend to downplay inborn temperament. The nature-nurture problem also has a political angle. Belief in the predominance of nature can be associated with conservatism, while belief in the predominance of nurture is often used to support the liberal view that human nature is highly malleable to changes in the environment.

Psychoanalysts have traditionally been wary of biological psychiatry. That is largely because they see it as deterministic. One of my psychoanalytic teachers said that if he were to believe that there were genetic factors in mental illness, he would feel hopeless. This was a mistake. Even if some theories favoring nature over nurture have been seen in that way, biological factors in development are not fixed for all time. For example, the relatively new discipline of *epigenetics* describes how switches related to environmental condition turn genes on and off (Carey, 2012). Moreover, most heritable traits are associated with small effects in hundreds of genes, while outcomes are only partially influenced by temperament, and are modified by life experiences (Rutter, 2006).

While biological and environmental theories of the mind differ in the extent to which human behavior is seen as deriving from genes or life experience, research shows that both play a role, and that pathological outcomes reflect an interaction between genes and environment (Rutter, 2006). Moreover, genetic variations affecting vulnerability to psychopathology can be adaptive under one set of circumstances, but maladaptive under another (Belsky and Pluess, 2009).

Psychoanalysts who see personality and psychopathology as primarily shaped by early experiences sometimes make the understanding of psychopathology into a detective story in which forgotten events from childhood turn out to be the culprit. That view is also mistaken. Whatever one's life experience, there are large individual differences in how people react to events. For this reason, the long-term effects of life adversities can only be understood in the context of temperament and genetic vulnerabilities (Rutter, 2006). The practical implication of this principle is that there can never be a "complete" analysis – only a method that helps people cope within the limits of their temperament. Moreover, in Freud's (1930) vision, human needs will always be in conflict with those of society.

But as psychoanalysis turned into a cause, "going into therapy" came to be recommended for every human problem. Adherents believed that the world would be a better place if everyone was treated. Melanie Klein even thought that if children were properly analyzed, neurotic symptoms could entirely disappear (Grosskurth, 1984).

One can still see these Utopian ideas reflected in popular advice columns that routinely advise "counseling" for every kind of problem. The idea that talking can heal life's ills also underlies the idea that every traumatic event (such as a massacre) requires immediate help from counselors. Ironically, research shows that early intervention for recently traumatized people can be damaging, and that it is usually better to avoid talking, at least for a while (Shalev, 2000). Moreover, most people exposed to adverse life events do not develop PTSD (McNally, 2003). Nonetheless, patients with a history of early adversity may be offered extensive courses of "trauma-based" therapy that are not really evidence-based.

Trauma and psychoanalysis

In the history of ideas, theories do not stand alone, but can be framed within a "*zeitgeist*" – a consensus view of the world that may be taken for granted, but that shapes every form of inquiry. In spite of Freud's doubts, psychoanalysis, with its focus on how childhood shapes the mind, has generally favored nurture over nature. It has sometimes misled therapists to search for culprits, usually the patient's parents. This is one of its weaknesses as a therapy. It has never been shown in empirical research that remembering or working through past events (and/or linked to the transference), is a reliable cure for psychological symptoms.

Sometimes the search for early trauma as an explanation of psychopathology goes back to infancy. One example was the theory that autism is due to "refrigerator mothers". This idea, originally suggested by the psychiatrist Leo Kanner (1943), was later elaborated by Bruno Bettelheim (1967), who claimed that autistic children were only trying to escape parents who had mistreated them. This idea, which many at the time took seriously, was a terrible disservice to autistic children and to their families (Pollak, 1997).

A second example was the theory that psychosis is due to "schizophrenogenic" mothering (Fromm-Reichmann, 1954). This idea, promoted by a group of American psychoanalysts, was scientifically invalid, and did real damage to patients whose psychoses could not be cured by psychotherapy, as well as to families who were blamed for a tragic illness for which they were not responsible (Dolnick, 1998).

A third example is the idea that borderline personality disorder is due to sexual abuse during childhood (Herman et al., 1989). While it is true that childhood abuse is common in BPD, and is a risk factor for the disorder, most patients have not suffered from significant abuse of this kind (Paris, 2008). A better way of understanding BPD is as an interaction between temperamental vulnerability and family dysfunction, which is as likely to take the form of emotional neglect as of abuse (Laporte et al., 2011).

A fourth example is the scandal that emerged 20 years ago over "recovered memories" of trauma in psychotherapy patients. This issue underlines how an excessive focus on childhood trauma can compromise the practice of psychotherapy. This story, which had major reverberations in society, and still does, deserves detailed examination.

Trauma and recovered memories

One of the most dramatic examples in recent decades of an excessive focus on childhood trauma derives from the concept of "recovered memory". This idea can be traced back to the early days of psychoanalysis. *The* belief that repressed memories of trauma are a common cause of adult psychopathology was once influential, and some clinicians still hold that view. The assumption is that child abuse is much more common than anyone thinks, that memories of trauma are often repressed, and that severe psychological problems in adulthood are the result of these experiences (Herman, 1992).

A crucial mistake underlying the concept or recovered memories derived from Freud, who thought that the brain records every moment of life as it is lived, much like a videorecorder (Breuer and Freud, 1955). If you did not remember negative life events (most people cannot recall much before about age five), the explanation had to be *repression*. Freud also claimed that psychoanalysis could remove this repression, and, much like archeology, uncover the secrets of the past.

It is now widely understood that the brain is highly selective about which memories it retains on its "hard drive" (Schacter, 2001; McNally, 2003). Most life events are forgotten. Moreover, what we do remember is not particularly accurate, and is greatly influenced by more recent events (Lane et al., 2015). Thus, memory is not necessarily historically accurate, but is a creative retelling that is more like a story than a reliable record of events (Loftus and Ketcham, 1994). That is why courts should never rely on eyewitness testimony, which is all too often wrong, and why it is easy to create false memories and convince people they are true (Loftus, 1979). The reason for false memories is much the same as for false beliefs. They create a "narrative fallacy" in which history is organized into a story that is easy to remember, whether true or false. Unfortunately, too many psychotherapists have been ignorant of these scientific findings.

Twenty years ago, a fad developed for the exploration in psychotherapy of "recovered memories" of child abuse (McHugh, 2005), associated with the dubious diagnosis of multiple personality disorder, or dissociative identity disorder (Paris, 2012). It is true that children are abused more often than most people had previously thought (Fergusson and Mullen, 1999). But it is not true that such events are often forgotten – on the contrary, traumatic memories tend to be intrusive, and can continue to trouble people decades later. It is also not true that child abuse is a predictable cause of symptoms – fortunately, most children are resilient, particularly if later life events are more helpful than hurtful (Fergusson and Mullen, 1999). Finally, it is not true that one can assume a history of child abuse from any specific psychological problem.

These false beliefs caused great damage. Patients were encouraged to focus on imaginary injuries, at the expense of recovery. Families were torn apart by claims that parents had committed incest. Some patients were diagnosed with fictional conditions, such as multiple personality disorder, and treated with harmful therapy. And best-selling books, e.g. "The Courage to Heal", written by two teachers (Bass and Davis, 1988), convinced some people that if you don't remember traumatic events, that only proves that you must have been exposed to them.

This epidemic was greatly encouraged by the book "Sybil" (Schreiber, 1989), which told a dramatic story of abuse and "multiples" that was later shown to be a fabrication (Nathan, 2011). I remember reading excerpts in my local newspaper, and wondering why I never saw anything so interesting, not realizing I was the victim of a massive deception. Even worse, epidemics of false accusations of abuse occurred in day care centers, putting many innocent people in jail (McHugh, 2005).

How could this have happened? Mental health professionals are often thought of as unusually intelligent and reasonable. In fact, most therapists rejected these ideas, and did not participate in the fad. But quite a few did. Once they began to believe in the ubiquity of child abuse and its repression, there was no way back. Like members of a cult, they found reasons to see everything they perceived as confirmation of a false belief. With the best of intentions, they did serious harm. Even today, clinicians who believe in this story are taken seriously and write best-selling books (e.g., van der Kolk, 2014).

Twenty-five years ago, the McGill University psychiatry department invited Harold Lief, an American psychoanalyst with a specialty in sex education, to give two invited talks, the first a public lecture, and the second a talk for professionals. However, when publicity went out, some believers in the recovered memory movement became aware that Lief was an opponent, who did not accept that sexual abuse and incest were necessarily primary causes of mental illness. This group of believers (most of whom were not professionals) came to the public lecture with the intention of disrupting it. Lief was interrupted from the first few minutes of his talk by people with noise-makers; one of the protestors let loose a stink bomb. They then gained support from a psychologist from Ottawa who leapt to the podium, took the microphone, and began to explain why a lecture of this kind could not be permitted. The Dean of Medicine, who was present, called for academic freedom, but was shouted down, and the event had to be abandoned. The professional lecture at a local hospital the next day went ahead, but the police had to be called in for protection.

This hardly sounds like the academic environment one expects at a large university. (Of course, several recent incidents of this kind have been widely covered in the media, and are considered a threat to free speech on campus.) But the recovered memory movement was full of passion. Its belief was that girls and women were being constantly abused, and that psychiatry, ever since Freud, had played a role in covering up the truth. This was explosive stuff, and it made for drama and a kind of "guerilla theatre".

My research group has studied trauma in patients with borderline personality disorder (Paris et al., 1994), and found that about a third of our sample had histories of childhood sexual abuse that went beyond single molestations by strangers. While this number was high, the majority of cases could not be explained on that basis. Later research showed that sisters of these patients who had suffered the same abuse almost never developed BPD, and these differences in outcome were largely accounted for by personality trait profiles (Laporte et al., 2011). The idea that these patients, or their sisters, could have repressed any recollection of such events flies in the face of everything we know about trauma and memory (McNally, 2003).

Twenty years ago, I was invited to a Canadian university to participate in a conference on trauma. On arrival, I learned that a group of therapists in the city were deeply committed to the construct of multiple personality disorder, and to its treatment through the recovery of repressed memories of trauma. They believed that the patients with BPD that I was talking about must be victims of childhood sexual abuse. To my discomfort, I was paired with a psychologist who took precisely that position. At one point, I said that you could be sure if a memory was false if patients reported obviously fictional events such as "Satanic ritual abuse". You could hear an audible hiss coming from the true believers in the audience.

My conclusion after this event was that one cannot easily overcome emotional biases, particularly among true believers. Even in an academic forum it is difficult to address such controversial issues effectively. In the popular mind, ideas about recovered memory have had an almost irresistible fascination. A book promoting the theory that *most* psychological problems in women are due to repressed child abuse sold a million copies (Bass and Davis, 1988). These complex issues require less passion and detailed attention to research data. My best option was to write about recovered memory fad and the false belief in the existence of multiple personality and dissociative disorders (Paris, 2012).

The false beliefs to which mental health professionals fell victim during the "epidemic" of recovered memory were based on incorrect theoretical ideas. The sicker people were, the more sure were their therapists that they had suffered something terrible in their childhood. Moreover, psychotherapy, and the use of hypnosis, acted as powerful tools to evoke false memories (McNally, 2003). (These highly suggestive methods were originally used by Freud.)

Recovered memory is a dramatic theory, and Hollywood has made much use of it. (To consider one example, Alfred Hitchcock directed a 1945 film called "Spellbound", whose script was written making use of advice from a psychoanalyst.) However, the concept of repressed memories of trauma is entirely unscientific, as researchers have clearly shown. Today we hear little about such ideas, and they have become marginal. In the end, the only way to combat false beliefs affecting psychiatry was through scientific research that eventually pointed to the truth.

Research consistently shows that childhood trauma, even severe trauma, does not *necessarily* produce mental disorders (Fergusson and Mullen, 1999). The relationship is statistical, but not consistent, and is modulated by temperamental vulnerability. Moreover, by the mid-20th century, psychologists, such as the Harvard professor Gordon Allport (1963), had gathered evidence showing that present circumstances trump childhood experiences. By and large, while adverse early experiences increase the risk for psychopathology, the onset of mental disorders in adulthood is more related to recent events. This principle is now widely accepted, supported by a large body of research demonstrating the ubiquity if resilience to adversity (Rutter, 2006). There is, however, an issue of dosing: severe and persistent events are much more likely to produce vulnerability to later events than single episodes.

Yet even taking these complexities into account, a preference for nurture over nature (or vice versa, as is common in neuroscience) does not do justice to the multiple interacting factors that shape human development. One again, psychoanalysis could benefit by absorbing the implications of empirical research.

Nature, nurture, and the social sciences

In a classic book, *The Blank Slate*, the psychologist Steven Pinker (2002) described the tendency to favor nurture over nature as characteristic of what he called the "Standard Social Science Model". In that view, biology plays a very minor role in human nature, and psychological and social development are almost entirely the product of life experiences.

Pinker went on to describe two points of view on the human condition. One, a *tragic vision*, is that there is no perfection in life, only adaptation to the limitations of human nature. In contrast, a *Utopian vision* implies that perfectibility is possible, both for individuals and for society. Pinker saw the evidence as confirming a tragic vision, criticizing what he called a "Standard Social Science Model", which denied the existence of human nature, and viewed social conditions not as givens, but as problems that can be overcome. Pinker reviewed a large body of evidence, concluding that there is a universal human nature that can be modified, but not radically changed, by political or social reforms.

A Utopian vision of the human condition has been most influential in the social sciences. It lies behind the reluctance to accept biological constraints on individual behavior or on the structure of society. The idea, going back to the British philosopher John Locke (1690), is that since children are "blank slates", they can learn new ways of living from benign educators. This view contrasts with the position of another British philosopher, Thomas Hobbes, that strong governments are needed to suppress natural tendencies to anarchy. That view is more consistent with Freud's version of psychoanalysis. Pinker (2002) supported Hobbes, with the caveat that the idea that human beings were ever solitary is wrong; people have always been social, and there is no such thing as a "social contract".

Pinker gives an example of Hobbesian anarchy that I lived through myself – the Montreal police strike of 1969. The removal of external restraints, even for a day, was immediately followed by rioting and looting, requiring the government to call in the army to regain control.

Yet a high level of cooperation has always been part of the secret of human success as a species (Melis and Semmann, 2010). People can be either selfish or cooperative depending on circumstances. By and large, given a perception of fairness, most people prefer to cooperate. One can even see compassionate behavior in young children (Kagan and Lamb, 1990). But there is wide individual variation in cooperative behavior:

the most selfish among us are people against whom society will always require a defense (Shermer, 2015).

In summary, the social sciences have had much the same problem as psychology. By favoring nurture over nature, they fail to understand that human development is an interactional process in which both play a role.

Psychoanalysis and cultural anthropology

Psychoanalysis used to have a strong following in the social sciences. Clinical and developmental psychology were dominated by Freud's ideas for decades. But today as psychology, even in its clinical applications, aspires to be empirical, psychoanalysis has been marginalized. But as researchers have begun to evaluate its concepts empirically, this situation could change.

Cultural anthropology is the social science that most resembles psychoanalysis. Its tradition includes a method that resembles the use of clinical experience: *participant observation* (Jorgensen, 2015). Thus anthropologists do not use quantitative measurements but offer interpretations of cultures studied by a trained observer. In the past, Freud's ideas had a strong following in anthropology, and some analysts promoted his theories of child development to explain cultural differences (Kardiner, 1939).

The work of the German-American anthropologist, Franz Boas, and his student Margaret Mead, provides an illuminating parallel to the story of psychoanalysis. Using observational methods, and infused with theoretical biases, anthropologists came to some very doubtful conclusions.

Boas and Mead had argued for *cultural relativism* (Degler, 1991). They dismissed any theory of innate and universal human nature on the grounds that there was no cultural pattern without exceptions. The trick was to find some obscure island or tribe which few people had ever visited, and where life seems to proceed by different rules. People who read these books, having never been to the places described, had to believe that the observations of anthropologists were accurate – in spite of the fact that the authors were out to prove something and had a strong political agenda. Their methods resembled those used by psychoanalysis, in that they observed a few cultures, and came to very broad conclusions, often after only months of field work. Contemporary anthropologists take a more nuanced view of cultural differences, and emphasize universals (Brown, 1991). Yet these arguments had, and still have, a great influence on the educated public.

In a best-selling book, Mead (1928) claimed that adolescents growing up in Samoa enjoyed total sexual freedom, and were therefore happier than Americans of the same age. Her theoretical bias was largely based on Freud's theories about the impact of sexual repression, but also reflected her own "liberated" life style (Lutkehaus, 2003). But Mead got everything wrong – by projecting her own ideology and personal agenda on the women she interviewed. Mead was out to prove that Americans should live more like Samoans, and to indulge in sexual freedom (as she did).

Mead's attempt to show that Samoans were really "flappers" was widely believed. After all, Americans in the 1920s were in the process of changing their own sexual behavior. Mead also believed that Samoans were hardly ever violent, and what violence did occur was the result of colonialism. She seemed to believe that human nature was pacific, and that it had only been spoiled by civilization. These ideas were also influenced by psychoanalysis, in that they explained cultural deviations as due to parenting practices.

Mead became a public intellectual, writing for women's magazines about how to raise children. (In this era, a tendency to pontificate on this subject was also common among psychoanalysts.) Mead did not suffer much from being mistaken – or admit that she had ever been mistaken about anything. She spent only a few months on her field work, did not speak the language, and depended on young women who were her informants. Mead was unaware of data casting doubt on the concept of Samoa as a tropical paradise. (The painter Paul Gaugin had the same fantasy about Tahiti.) Many years later, an anthropologist who was actually an expert on Samoa, Derek Freeman, showed why Mead was wrong about sexual freedom among adolescents living in the South Pacific (Freeman, 1983). As in most human societies, adolescent sexuality in Samoa was tightly controlled to protect blood lines. He also showed that Samoa had much higher rates of rape and murder than North America. Freeman concluded that Mead had either made up much of her data, or primed her informants to provide what she wanted. But because of Mead's prestige, he only published this book after her death. The controversy continues even today, and Mead is still defended by those who hold on to her vision (Shankman, 2009).

I had the chance to meet Margaret Mead when a group of residents in psychiatry invited her to speak at one of a series of debates at McGill

University in 1972. Mead was clever but arrogant. When I picked her up at the airport she immediately criticized me for not arranging a VIP entrance through immigration. She felt much better when 500 people showed up for a debate on the impact of feminism on psychiatry. Mead, leaning on the shepherd's crook that she used in her later years, impressed everyone with her presence. The main idea of her talk was that children can be brought up outside traditional family settings, by women working together. Mead was right about that point – the sociobiologist Sara Hrdy (2011) later supported this hypothesis with solid data.

Mead had unusually high self-esteem. During her final illness in 1978, a nurse said to her, "But Dr. Mead, everyone has to die". Her reply was, "no, this is different" (Lutkehaus, 2003). Perhaps Mead suffered from the "acquired situational narcissism" that comes from constant adulation (Campbell et al., 2011).

Mead was typical of the intellectual climate of her time, sympathetic both to psychoanalysis and to left-wing politics. She may be best remembered for reviving the 18th-century concept of a "noble savage", uncorrupted by modern society. In this view, people are good until society makes them bad. Mead's assumption that people are happier in pre-modern societies is reminiscent of another common idea that children are innocent. (That idea must have been thought up by people who never been parents!) It is a contemporary version of Genesis, an expulsion from Eden that leaves behind memories of a lost paradise. Mead also considered human nature to be "unbelievably malleable" (Mead, 1935). To his credit, Sigmund Freud did not share that illusion.

Biology may not determine how we live our lives, but it defines the *constraints* on human possibilities. The idea that humans are infinitely malleable is unscientific and potentially dangerous. (It was also the basis of "scientific socialism", a movement that has suffered an even stepper decline than has classical psychoanalysis.) To make psychoanalytic therapy truly scientific, we need to recognize the limitations of the model and be humble in the face of contrary evidence.

Genes, neuroscience, and human nature

In recent years, with the rise of neuroscience, the emphasis on nurture in intellectual circles has been reversed. People are now more impressed with the findings of genetics and molecular biology.

Some of the data contradicting the standard social science model comes from research in *behavioral genetics* (the study of similarities and differences between identical and non-identical twins). Identical twins are more similar than fraternal twins, so that almost all traits have a heritable component of about 50% (Plomin et al., 2013). This does not mean that "everything is genetic"; 50% of the variance is still shaped by the environment. Moreover, genes interact with the environment during development; the recently developed field of epigenetics (Carey, 2012) has shown that gene expression is modified by environmental events. In light of these (and many other) findings, the climate of opinion in psychology in the 21st century has undergone a sea change.

The Harvard developmental psychologist Jerome Kagan (2006) has written about his intellectual development in a zeitgeist dominated by childhood determinism, in which everyone took psychoanalysis more or less for granted. Like many intellectuals of his generation, since he believed in a better world, he wanted to believe that if nurture is everything, then everything can be changed. It was only when Kagan's own research into inborn temperament in children contradicted these assumptions that he changed his mind – as any good scientist should do.

Judith Rich Harris, author of several textbooks in developmental psychology, had a similar intellectual journey, becoming a convert from childhood determinism to behavioral genetics. Harris (1998) published a best-seller, "The Nurture Assumption" that challenged many of the previous assumptions of her field, i.e., that parenting is the main determinant of personality, intelligence, and mental health. It was notable for the way she used science to release parents from the accusation that whatever was wrong with their children must be their fault. The evidence reviewed by Harris showed that twin studies demonstrate that growing up in the same family does not make children similar, and that genes play a much greater role in shaping adult personality and functioning than most people believe. These principles have been conclusively demonstrated in many behavioral genetic studies.

For her heresy, Harris was attacked by many social scientists. Today her ideas lie in the scientific mainstream. Harris never said that "everything is genetic". Her point was that the impact of life experience depends on temperament. The same events will produce completely different effects in different people. These ideas have been consistently supported by research. Later, Harris (2006) went on to argue that social forces, acting largely through peer groups, are at least as important as family life in the development of personality.

Sociobiology is a discipline developed by the Harvard biologist Edward O. Wilson (1975), now usually termed *evolutionary psychology*. This research has presented evidence that natural selection not only shapes anatomy and physiology, but also plays a major role in human behavior. In "The Selfish Gene", Richard Dawkins (1976) proposed that the gene, and not the individual or the group, is the basic unit of natural selection. These ideas are now highly influential, even if they still spark controversy.

One might think that the concept that people have a biological nature would be unexceptionable. Why should the brain be different from any other organ in the body? Yet sociobiology met a furious attack from many scientists. Two Harvard biology professors (both Marxists), Steven Jay Gould and Richard Lewontin, argued that the brain had no specific behavioral programs determined by natural selection, but could be thought of as an all-purpose organ, designed to make best use of its environment (Lewontin et al., 1990). But as a leading American biologist, Theodosius Dobzhansky (1964), once stated, "nothing in biology makes sense without evolution". Evolutionary psychology sees the brain as a kind of Swiss army knife, with a variety of tools, each designed for a specific purpose. But the biological universals in human nature are not "blueprints", but general guidelines that vary from one individual to another.

These examples show that psychoanalysis is not alone in having problems with a fusion between biological and social thought. Its future requires the field to be open to input from research in other disciplines. What is needed is a biopsychosocial model in which temperament, life experience, and social forces all play a role in shaping personality and psychological symptoms. Neither is the idea that children are blank slates on which the environment makes its imprint. One new direction in research that could shape the future is epigenetics (Carey, 2012), in which gene expression is modified by environmental events.

Psychoanalysis still has the opportunity to join with other branches of psychology to discover the developmental pathways that make people what they are. They mechanisms will always be multivariate, not univariate. Applying an approach that takes complexity into account, the conflict between nature and nurture in psychological development could eventually have a happy (and integrative) ending.

References

Allport, G.: *Pattern and Growth in Personality*. San Diego, CA, Harcourt College Publishing, 1963.

Bass, E., Davis, L.: *The Courage to Heal*. New York, Greenwood, 1988.

Belsky, J., Pluess, M.: Beyond diathesis stress: Differential susceptibility to environmental influences. *Psychological Bulletin* 2009, 135: 885–908.

Bettelheim, B.: *The Empty Fortress: Infantile Autism and the Birth of the Self*. New York, Free Press, 1967.

Breuer, J., Freud, S.: Studies on Hysteria. In *The Standard Edition of the Complete Psychological Works of Sigmund Freud*, Volume 2. London, Hogarth Press, 1955.

Brown, D.E.: Human Universals. New York, McGraw Hill, 1991.

Campbell, W.K., Hoffman, B.J., Campbell, S.M., Marchisio, G.: Narcissism in organizational contexts. *Human Resource Management Review* 2011, 21: 268–284.

Carey, N.: *The Epigenetic Revolution*. New York, Columbia University Press, 2012.

Dawkins, R.: *The Selfish Gene*. Oxford, Oxford University Press, 1976.

Degler, C.N.: *In Search of Human Nature: The Decline and Revival of Darwinism in American Social Thought*. New York, Oxford University Press, 1991.

Dobzhansky, T.: Biology: Molecular and organismic. *American Zoologist* 1964, 35: 125–129.

Dolnick, E.: *Madness on the Couch: Blaming the Victim in the Heyday of Psychoanalysis*. New York, Simon and Schuster, 1998.

Fergusson, D.M., Mullen, P.E.: *Childhood Sexual Abuse: An Evidence Based Perspective*. Thousand Oaks, CA, Sage Publications, 1999.

Freeman, D.: *Margaret Mead and Samoa*. Cambridge, MA, Harvard University Press, 1983.

Freud, S.: *Civilization and Its Discontents*. New York, Norton, 1930/1989.

Fromm-Reichmann, F.: Psychotherapy of schizophrenia. *American Journal of Psychiatry* 1954, 111: 410–415.

Grosskurth, P.: *Melanie Klein: Her World and Her Work*. New York, Knopf, 1984.

Harris, J.R.: *The Nurture Assumption*. New York, Free Press, 1998.

Harris, J.R.: *No Two Alike: Human Nature and Human Individuality*. New York, Norton, 2006.

Herman, J.L., Perry, J.C., van der Kolk, B.A.: Childhood trauma in borderline personality disorder. *American Journal of Psychiatry* 1989, 146: 490–495.

Herman, J.L.: *Trauma and Recovery*. New York, Basic Books, 1992.

Hrdy, S.B.: *Mothers and Others the Evolutionary Origins of Mutual Understanding*. Cambridge, MA, Harvard University Press, 2011.

Jorgensen, D.L.: *Participant Observation*. London, Wiley, 2015.

Kagan, J.: *An Argument for Mind*. New Haven, Yale University Press, 2006.

Kagan, J., Lamb, S., eds.: *The Emergence of Morality in Young Children*. Chicago, University of Chicago Press, 1990.

Kanner, L.: Autistic disturbances of affective contact. *The Nervous Child* 1943, 2: 217–250.

Kardiner, A.: *The Individual and His Society: The Psychodynamics of Primitive Social Organization*. New York, Columbia University Press, 1939.

Lane, R.D., Ryan, L., Nadel, L., Greenberg, L.: Memory reconsolidation, emotional arousal, and the process of change in psychotherapy: New insights from brain science. *Behavioral and Brain Sciences* 2015, 38: 1–80.

Laporte, L., Paris, J., Russell, J., Guttman, H.: Psychopathology, trauma, and personality traits in patients with borderline personality disorder and their sisters. *Journal of Personality Disorders* 2011, 25: 448–462.
Lewontin, R., Rose, S., Kamin, L.: *Not in Our Genes: Biology, Ideology and Human Nature*. London, Penguin Books, 1990.
Locke, J.: *An Essay Concerning Human Understanding*, 1st edition, 1 vols. London, Thomas Bassett, 1690.
Loftus, E.F.: *Eyewitness Testimony*. Cambridge, MA, Harvard University Press, 1979.
Loftus, E.F., Ketcham, K.: *The Myth of Repressed Memory*. New York, St. Martin's Press, 1994.
Lutkehaus, N.: *Margaret Mead: The Making of an American Icon*. Princeton, Princeton University Press, 2003.
McHugh, P.R.: The Mind Has Mountains. Baltimore, Johns Hopkins Press, 2005.
McNally, R.L.: *Remembering Trauma*. Cambridge, MA, Harvard University Press, 2003.
Mead, M.: *Coming of Age in Samoa: A Psychological Study of Primitive Youth for Western Civilization*. New York, Perennial Classics, 1928/2001.
Mead, M.: *Sex and Temperament in Three Primitive Societies*. New York, Morrow, 1935.
Melis, A.P., Semmann, D.: How is human cooperation different? *Philosophical Transactions of the Royal Society of Biological Sciences* 2010, 365: 2663–2774.
Nathan, D.: *Sibyl Exposed*. New York, Simon and Schuster, 2011.
Paris, J.: *Treatment of Borderline Personality Disorder*. New York, Guilford Press, 2008.
Paris, J.: The rise and fall of dissociative disorders. *Journal of Nervous and Mental Diseases* 2012, 200: 1076–1079.
Paris, J., Zweig-Frank, H., Guzder, J.: Psychological risk factors for borderline personality disorder in female patients. *Comprehensive Psychiatry* 1994, 35: 301–305.
Pinker, S.: *The Blank Slate: The Modern Denial of Human Nature*. New York, Viking, 2002.
Plomin, R., DeFries, J.C., Knopik, V.S., Neiderhiser, J.N.: *Behavioral Genetics*, 6th edition. New York, Palgrave MacMillan, 2013.
Pollak, R.: *The Creation of Dr. B: A Biography of Bruno Bettelheim*. New York, Touchstone, 1997.
Rutter, M.J.: *Genes and Behavior: Nature-Nurture Interplay Explained*. London, Blackwell, 2006.
Schacter, D.: *The Seven Sins of Memory*. New York, Houghton Mifflin, 2001.
Schreiber, F.: *Sybil: The Classic True Story of a Woman Possessed by Sixteen Personalities*. New York, Grand Central, 1989.
Shalev, A.Y.: Treating survivors in the immediate aftermath of traumatic events. In R. Yehuda, ed.: *Treating Trauma Survivors with PTSD*. Washington, DC, American Psychiatric Publishing, 2000, pp. 157–188.
Shankman, P.: *The Trashing of Margaret Mead*. Madison, University of Wisconsin Press, 2009.
Shermer, M.: *The Moral Arc: How Science and Reason Lead Us to Truth*. New York, Holt, 2015.
Van der Kolk, B.: *The Body Keeps the Score: Brain, Mind, and Body in the Healing of Trauma*. New York, Penguin, 2014.
Wilson, E.O.: *Sociobiology: The New Synthesis*. Cambridge, MA, Harvard University Press, 1975.

Chapter 8

Psychoanalysis beyond the clinic

In this chapter, we move beyond the clinic, as well as beyond the boundaries of science. The relationship of psychoanalysis to humanistic disciplines and to the less rigorous social sciences is of some interest, but it is not subject to empirical investigation. We therefore have to consider ideas that are plausible, but that cannot be considered as provable by scientific methods.

Psychoanalysis and the humanities

Psychoanalysis, which can be understood as a sub-discipline of psychology, has also had an influence on disciplines far beyond clinical settings. As it became less central to psychiatry and psychology, psychoanalysis found a new home in the humanities (Elliott and Prager, 2016). This was not a new development. Freud had tried his hand on applying psychoanalysis to biography, as well as to history, literature, and culture (Schultz, 2005). Literary critics have long been fascinated with Freud's ideas, applying them to the understanding of authors and/or their fictional characters (Adams and Szaluta, 1996).

For example, *psychohistory* and *psychobiography* attempted to explain historical developments and the trajectory of lives by examining childhood experiences, or by parenting practices within a given culture (DeMause, 1982; Lifton, 1986). A recent special issue of *Psychoanalytic Psychology* was devoted to psychohistory (Roth, 2016). However, this approach has been criticized for finding causal relationships based on psychological data alone (Stannard, 1982). The problem with the methods of such hybrid disciplines is that historical forces are very distant from the psychological mechanisms used to understand individuals. It is difficult to see how cultural and social phenomena can be accounted for in a meaningful way by intrapsychic forces, or by the quality of interpersonal relationships. The problem is, as is the case for explaining psychopathology, that for every person with a difficult childhood or a dysfunctional family, there are many others who are resilient and do well in life (see Chapter 5). For this reason, an emphasis on childhood trauma without considering that many or most children have similar experiences, has led psychobiography to be criticized as "pathography" (Wiltshire, 2000).

Post-modernism and psychoanalysis

In the last several decades, some scholars have fitted psychoanalytic theory into a program of *post-modernism*, an influential set of ideas that shapes much of current thought in the humanities (Harvey, 1990; Phillips, 1991). Post-modernism has been defined in many ways, but its core idea is that there is no such thing as universal truth, and that claims to knowledge are socially constructed. The idea that truth is always relative rather than absolute is clearly anti-science. This idea can be considered as form of counter-enlightenment, a struggle against the primary of reason (Pinker, 2018). Moreover, denying the existence of truth should make the claims of post-modernist theorists equally doubtful of their own ideas. However the pet theories held by these writers are rarely subjected to the same "deconstruction".

Post-modern ideas have been adopted to create a new form of literary criticism that draws ideas from psychoanalysis, Marxism, feminism, and post-structuralism (Selden et al., 2005). By and large, the movement is strong on rhetoric and weak on data.

While few practicing analysts would describe themselves as post-modernists, these interfaces were the subject of a special issue of *Psychoanalytic Inquiry* (Citaravese et al., 2015). Freud's ideas, rooted in 19th-century philosophy, are not in any way consistent with post-modernism, which denies the value of science (Bell, 2009). The application of post-modernism to psychoanalysis would move the field even further away from empiricism. Some analysts have taken a "hermeneutic" position (Ricoeur, 1981), following Nietzche's dictum that there are no facts, only interpretations. Unfortunately, doing so only creates a license for speculation: post-modernists have a worrying tendency of relying on glib but unproven assumptions.

That is precisely the problem with the ideas of the French philosopher Michel Foucault (1982), who argued that all claims for truth only hide a quest for power. I have struggled to understand why such a shallow thinker became one of the most quoted writers in the history of intellectual thought. Again, the idea that truth does not exist is self-contradictory – post-modernists should be no more believable than anyone else. Crucially, Foucault was entirely hostile to the scientific enterprise and dismissed research findings of any kind. Yet Foucault's ideas have strongly influenced the development of "critical theory", an offshoot of Marxism that attempts to use literary criticism as a way of reforming society (Geuss, 1981).

I read "Madness and Civilization" (Foucault, 1965) as a psychiatric resident, but only realized later how far the author deviated from historical facts, making the incorrect claim that people with psychosis were treated well in pre-modern societies (Shorter, 1997). Moreover, Foucault was one of a group of French philosophers who are responsible for the obscurity and unreadability of so many post-modern books and articles in the last few decades. His highly verbose discourse is difficult to penetrate, but this difficulty may have made him more popular among academics. Finally, Foucault was far from alone in rejecting science, and this position could be used to protect speculative ideas from scientific scrutiny.

For the last 40 years, there has been intense interest among humanists in the ideas of the French psychoanalyst Jacques Lacan (2001). Lacan formed his own "school" in France, separate from mainstream psychoanalytic societies, claiming that he was carrying out "a return to Freud" (Roudinesco, 1990). This claim was not true – except in the sense that Lacan was even more speculative than Freud, and had much less interest in scientific data. Even so, Lacan's theories became "the latest thing" in psychoanalysis for many humanist scholars, and stimulated many books (Google Scholar currently lists over 600). But there has never been empirical research on any of the constructs that Lacan proposed.

Lacan's writings are difficult to summarize, given that they are even more obscure and impenetrable than Foucault's. While some of his constructs have their roots in post-war Parisian intellectual life, they use idiosyncratic terminology, such as "mirror stage", "desire", or "signifiers" (Roudinesco, 1990). Without any training in mathematics, Lacan even attempted to integrate some of its advanced concepts into his theory

(Sokal and Bricmont, 1998). Clearly Lacan never felt a need to tame his hubris.

Another point of contention was Lacan's use of a "variable length session", which gave up the 50-minute hour in favor of sessions that could last for only a few minutes (and were sometimes held in a taxi). Lacan became a millionaire as a result of getting patients to accept brief sessions, and had no compunction about having sex with some of his patients (Roudinesco, 1990). The British philosopher and author Dylan Evans (2005, p. 40), who was also trained as an analyst, described his disillusionment with Lacan as follows:

> As I became more familiar with Lacan's teachings, the internal contradictions and lack of external confirmation became ever more apparent. And as I tried to make sense of Lacan's bizarre rhetoric, it became clearer to me that the obfuscatory language did not hide a deeper meaning, but was in fact a direct manifestation of the confusion inherent in Lacan's own thought.

The British author and critic of psychoanalysis, Richard Webster (2017), describes a similar reaction to Lacan's movement:

> The Lacan phenomenon is a bizarre one. Attempts to understand it have not been helped by the insistence of many of Lacan's apologists that the "pure" theoretical issues can be separated from Lacan's therapeutic practice and the extraordinary manner in which he behaves towards his disciples. Such an attitude is no more defensible in the case of Lacan than it is in the case of Freud himself. Indeed, perhaps the only real resemblance between Lacan and Freud is that both played the role of prophet or messiah with extraordinary effectiveness and both attracted disciples who treated their person as sacred and their word as law.

As Chomsky (2013) observed, Lacan was in most ways a charlatan. The puzzle is how his thought became an international movement that fascinated many intelligent people. (The same question could be raised about scientology, or any other unscientific but popular system of belief.) What is also puzzling is that almost four decades after his death, there is still a fad for Lacanian ideas among humanists. Like Foucault, Lacan presented himself as a heroic dissident, and appealed to those who love words more than science. But obscurity does not create profundity. While many books have been inspired by the ideas of Lacan, few psychoanalysts (outside of France) have incorporated them into their practice. One has to wonder whether ideas can be adopted *because* of their obscurity, and if they are promulgated by guru-like figures.

In summary, post-modernism has nothing positive to contribute to psychoanalysis or psychology. The rejection of empiricism is a move backwards, not forwards. Yes, truth, particularly about the mind is hard to determine. But idealizing speculation can do nothing to help psychoanalysis integrate with science.

Psychoanalysis and feminism

The most productive relationship between psychoanalysis and the humanities may be its dialogue with feminism. It is no secret that Freud's views about women were patriarchal and out of date. Even if he invited many female analysts to join his movement, the classical forms of analysis did not understand women very well. Overall, Freud's formulations centered on male psychology, and failed to take a relational perspective.

Today it would be surprising to find analysts who still believe that women can only find fulfillment through having children and caring for their families. But the American cultural tradition encourages women to be more independent than their counterparts in other parts of the world. This is also where psychoanalysis had its strongest following (Samuel, 2013).

Since the 1970s, a meeting ground between psychoanalysis and feminism has become possible. Among others, the New Zealand-born British analyst Juliet Mitchell (1974) was a pioneering voice. In part, the shift from the drive theories of classical psychoanalysis and modern relational theories reflects the influence of feminism.

As is the case for all revisions of the psychoanalytic model, there has been no research to determine whether feminist principles make analytic methods of treatment more effective. But the analytic movement would have suffered greatly if it had not taken on the cause of equality for women. However, this development needs to be seen separate from post-modernism, which is obsessed with gender, and with removing gender as a meaningful category in human psychology.

Psychoanalysis and Marxism

One might think that psychoanalysis and Marxism are incompatible. After all psychoanalysis favors individual freedom and is based on introspection, while Marxism favors social change and advises activism. Yet both these ideas appeared at the end of the 19th and the beginning of the 20th century, a time when traditional values and religious systems were in decline, and when people were looking for meaning in new ways (Zaretsky, 2004).

One of the more serious efforts to link these paradigms was developed by the Frankfurt school political scientist Herbert Marcuse (1956). This was a Utopian vision of a society that provided material equality and that eliminated sexual repression entirely. These fantastic ideas were hardly practical, but they had a certain influence on the counter-culture during the 1960s. Later, they were absorbed into post-modernism and the political tradition of the New Left (Zaretsky, 2016).

But while every analyst has his or her own political views, it is hard to see how Marxism can influence the way that therapy is conducted. The same can be said for religious beliefs, which rarely play any part in psychoanalysis. By and large, effective psychological treatment encourages patients to take responsibility for their own lives, and not to blame problems on society.

Psychoanalysis, society, and narcissism

Sociologists who have applied psychoanalytic principles to the study of sociology have been particularly interested in the problem of narcissism. While psychoanalysis has been used to modify narcissism in patients, it may also promote it by encouraging people to put their own needs ahead of social obligations.

The American historian Christopher Lasch (1979) wrote an influential book in which he argued that narcissism was no longer a problem for individuals, but for the culture at large. While this view was based on his own impressions, it was confirmed later by research using standard measure of narcissistic traits (Twenge and Campbell, 2009). This evidence suggests that young people are more likely to endorse narcissism on questionnaires, to have grandiose ideas, and to feel entitled to special treatment in life. But unlike Kohut, these researchers attribute this trend to the idea that children should be encouraged to have self-esteem, and that parents and teachers should make everyone feel special. This is a very American phenomenon, and reflects a culture that encourages people to feel that everything in life is possible. But it is doubtful that Sigmund Freud, with his darker view of human nature, would have agreed.

Therapy culture

The psychoanalytic movement found a cultural niche under specific cultural and historical conditions (Hale, 1995; Zaretsky, 2004). The rise of modernity in Western countries was characterized by a decline of traditional society and shared beliefs, favoring the individual over the collective. The decline of organized religion was associated with a loss of ultimate meaning. Psychological theories offer a new way of understanding the world, bringing order to the chaotic and complex demands of modern life, but sometimes had unfortunate side effects (Paris, 2012). Over 50 years ago, Rieff (1966) commented on the primacy of a therapeutic view of the human condition, noting that this could imply that people are not really responsible for their misdeeds.

"*Therapy culture*", a concept developed by the sociologist Frank Furedi (2004), describes how psychoanalytic ideas have become widely held assumptions, particularly among educated people. The term refers not just to therapy itself, but to ideologies derived from therapy, influencing how we view ourselves, how we live our lives, and how we raise our children. As the poet WH Auden wrote in an elegy on the death of Freud, "for us, he has now become, not a person, but a climate of opinion".

The principle that psychological problems are caused by childhood experiences led some parents to worry that they may damage their children. This tendency has been called "paranoid parenting" (Furedi, 2004).

The stance in which parents are blamed for psychological problems is a key feature of therapy culture. When parenting is based on irrational fears, it may not encourage autonomy in children. Some parents have even felt afraid to discipline or criticize their children, for fear that doing so might turn out to be "traumatic". A few parents have even been reluctant to let their children sleep in cribs, or to send them to day care, for fear of interfering with the attachment process. Yet research shows that differences between children in and out of day care are too small to be of any clinical significance. Moreover, children throughout history have usually been raised by multiple caretakers, not by one mother alone (Hrdy, 2011). But concern about inadequate attachment may have negatively affected contemporary parenting practices. In large-scale surveys, Twenge (2017), using survey data, documented some of the consequences of the current overprotective style of raising children in contemporary culture, which, combined with constant access to social media, may be making adolescents more anxious and (paradoxically) less social.

Unfortunately, the blaming of parents for psychological sometimes provides troubled people with unhelpful excuses. Patients in talking therapy can spend years exploring their feelings of deprivation in childhood, but do little or nothing to change their present life. Most therapists will have seen patients who detail every injury, large or small, that they have endured. But they would rather "talk the talk" than "walk the walk". Moreover, even if we all have an "inner child", we do not need to listen to it. (Some wags have even suggested that inner children can benefit from being sent to their rooms.)

Popular movements, such as those for recovery and self-help, have also promulgated a dogma of parental blame. The principle that "dysfunctional families" are psychologically crippling is widely accepted in our culture. And, as described in Chapter 7, some therapists have invented stories to place blame by encouraging false memories of child abuse, which have been used to account for every psychological problem.

Psychoanalysis creates a *narrative*, not a factually accurate exploration of a life history. Treating the past as the key determinant of current experience *seems* to offer a meaningful story. But this historical point of view leads to a paradox. The rights and wrongs of the present can be influenced by the past, but are not *determined* by it.

A more productive approach to psychotherapy could be based on the famous quip: "This is the first day of the rest of your life". The cognitive psychologist Marsha Linehan (1993) wisely advises patients to deal with parental failings and past traumatic events, not by trying to "work them through", but by "radical acceptance", i.e., moving on.

As clinicians well know, acceptance can be difficult. And as Alcoholics Anonymous has usefully put it, recovery occurs "one day at a time". Yet even the worst turns of fate can create opportunities to improve one's quality of life. We need only ask therapists who work with the chronically ill, or in palliative care for the dying. And in the end, while understanding life stories is essential, explaining current problems entirely on the basis of the past is illusory. Psychopathology emerges from a complex interaction between temperament, life experience, and the social environment.

Attributions of direct causality to childhood events are simplistic and not justified by empirical research.

Moreover, blaming others makes it easier to feel like a *victim*. Espousing a victim narrative, either from one's own experience, or from society at large (as supported by post-modernist thought), is not a pathway to psychological autonomy and ownership.

To move beyond a closed circle of self, people need to become responsible for their own lives. The ethos of talking therapy has encouraged people to see themselves as a victim of childhood experiences and past traumas. Therapeutic narratives that focus on an injured self can create a perception of having innocently suffered from the actions of others. This story rarely raises one's quality of life. Instead, it tends to confirm one's victimization (Dineen, 1996). These dramas have been widely played out in the media. Stories of trauma invite us to feel sorrow, pity, and anger – rather than admire resilience to adversity. A more positive identity for an adult with a truly traumatic past could be to define oneself as a "survivor".

Needless to say, psychotherapists must still "bear witness" to patients' life stories and deepest sorrows. Having someone "feel your pain" can be an important first step for helping people who have long felt misunderstood and invalidated. But that does not mean that patients need to spend *most* of the time in therapy talking about their childhood. Most people experience helpless feelings as children, but most are resilient to adversity, growing into adults who have choices and can choose to live differently (Rutter, 2007). No matter how difficult the past has been, there is no reason to remain in a victim role. Too much of a focus on past suffering encourages self-absorption and a sense of entitlement in the present.

This having been said, the past can certainly cast a shadow on the present. Research has generally confirmed the principle that past experiences make us more sensitive to situations that remind us of earlier difficulties (Rutter and Rutter, 1993). But these relationships are much more complicated than most therapists think. For example, past experiences can lead people to *choose* situations that are similar to the past, or to attempt to find situations that are the very opposite of the past. Life histories are important, but by no means deterministic.

Research has also documented a relationship between taking a victim role and narcissistic personality traits (McCullough et al., 2003). This makes sense, given that excessive self-regard can be supported by blaming others for failings. Yet a wide body of research shows that when something traumatic has happened, people need (as much as possible) to take control and achieve personal mastery (Infurna et al., 2015). One need not be mired in the past if there are options in the present.

Several aspects of modern culture encourage people to take on the victim role. Entire groups claim to become “empowered” by proclaiming their injuries. Autobiographies, which used to tell stories about conquering adversity through persistence and hard work, may now focus on the impact of adversity. Yet even people who have been subjected to the worst experiences (such as concentration camps) can rise above them and begin life again (Shrira et al., 2010). Moreover, most people who suffer childhood trauma grow up to be functioning adults (Paris, 2000). It is fortunate that human beings are resilient. If they were not, our species might have never survived.

Paradoxically, the status of victim gives some people an identity and a purpose. Experienced psychotherapists may begin by partially validating these perceptions, but encourage patients to move on. The principle is that people need to “own” their problems rather than feeling victimized by them. Otherwise, much like a traditional religious person invoking “God’s will”, patients can feel paralyzed by fate. The dialectic that drives therapy is to validate people’s life experiences – and then ask them to change. The process need not be disempowering. What one can say to patients is, “You have had a difficult time. But nothing prevents you now from making your life better”. This is much the same idea as “radical acceptance”.

Therapy culture follows Freud in seeing troubled people as victims of traumatic events, minimizing the agency they need to manage their lives. In fact, “therapizing” the human condition can distract people from their real problems. I once asked a physician who had worked in Ethiopia after its famine whether the survivors had PTSD, and was told, “they had no time for that”. Reality contradicted the idea that therapy is always needed to deal with trauma.

Even Freud spoke of converting neurotic misery into normal unhappiness (Breuer and Freud, 1955). Therapy culture, as well as in interminable treatments, runs the risk of giving people the impression that childhood trauma is a curse that can only be overcome by years of treatment. It derives from the same ideas that have threatened to make psychoanalysis interminable. These ideas are not supported by scientific evidence: most people who suffer trauma, either in childhood or later in life, do not develop mental disorders (Rutter, 2012). Even if everyone has a breaking point, human beings are built to be resilient.

Conclusion

Psychoanalysis is a part of modern life, and its vocabulary has entered common parlance. Along with other forms of psychotherapy, it has changed the way people think about human nature and motivation.

But psychoanalysis is not an all-embracing theory of the human condition. The transfer of psychoanalytic ideas from the clinic to the wider culture has sometimes been used to promote glib and simplistic explanations of a wide variety of cultural phenomena.

References

Adams, L., Szaluta, J., eds.: *Psychoanalysis and the Humanities*. New York, Psychology Press, 1996.

Bell, D.: Is truth an illusion? Psychoanalysis and postmodernism. *International Journal of Psychoanalysis* 2009, 90: 331–345.

Breuer, J., Freud, S: Studies in Hysteria. In J. Strachey, ed.: *The Standard Edition of the Complete Psychological Works of Sigmund Freud*, Volume 2, xxxii. London, Hogarth Press, 1955, originally published, 1895, pp. 1–335.

Chomsky, N.: Quoted in www.critical-theory.com/noam-chomsky-calls-jacques-lacan-a-charlatan/2013.

Citaravese, G., Katz, S.M., Tubert-Oaklander, J.: Prologue: Postmodernism and psychoanalysis. *Psychoanalytic Inquiry* 2015, 35: 559–565.

DeMause, L.: *Foundations of Psychohistory*. London, UK, Creative Roots Publishing, 1982.

Dineen, T.: *Manufacturing Victims: What the Psychology Industry Is Doing to People*. Westmount, Canada, Robert Davies, 1996.

Elliott, A., Prager, J.: *Routledge Handbook of Psychoanalysis in the Social Sciences and Humanities*. London, Routledge, 2016.

Evans, D.: From Lacan to Darwin. In J. Gottschall, D.S. Wilson, eds.: *The Literary Animal: Evolution and the Nature of Narrative*. Evanston, Northwestern University Press, 2005, pp. 38–55.

Foucault, M.: *Madness and Civilization*. New York, Vintage, 1965.

Foucault, M.: The subject and power. *Critical Inquiry* 1982, 8: 777–795.

Furedi, F.: *Therapy Culture: Cultivating Vulnerability in an Uncertain Age*. London, Routledge, 2004

Geuss, R.: *The Idea of a Critical Theory*. Cambridge, Cambridge University Press, 1981, from year one of IAPT, *Behaviour Research and Therapy* 51: 597e606.

Hale, R.: *The Rise and Crisis of Psychoanalysis in the United States*. New York, Oxford University Press, 1995.

Harvey, D.: *The Condition of Postmodernity*. Oxford, Wiley-Blackwell, 1990.

Hrdy, S.B.: *Mothers and Others the Evolutionary Origins of Mutual Understanding*. Cambridge, MA, Harvard University Press, 2011.

Infurna, F.J., Rivers, C.T., Reich, J., Zautra, A.J.: Childhood trauma and personal mastery: Their influence on emotional reactivity to everyday events in a community sample of middle-aged adults. *PLoS One* 2015, 10: e0121840.

Lacan, J.: *Ecrits: A Selection*. New York, Norton, 2001.

Lasch, C.: *The Culture of Narcissism*. New York, Warner, 1979.

Lifton, R.J.: *The Nazi Doctors: Medical Killing and the Psychology of Genocide*. New York, Basic Books, 1986.

Linehan, M.: *Cognitive Behavioral Therapy for Borderline Personality Disorder*. New York, Guilford Press, 1993.

Marcuse, H.: *Eros and Civilization: A Philosophical Inquiry into Freud*. London, UK, Routledge/Kegan Paul, 1956.

McCullough, M.E., Emmons, R.A., Kilpatrick, S.D.: Narcissists as "victims": The role of narcissism in the perception of transgressions. *Personality and Social Psychology Bulletin* 2003, 29: 885–893.

Mitchell, J.: *Psychoanalysis and Feminism: Freud, Reich, Laing, and Women*. New York, Pantheon Books, 1974.

Paris, J.: *Myths of Childhood*. Philadelphia, Brunner/Mazel, 2000.

Paris, J.: *Psychotherapy in an Age of Narcissism*. London, UK, Palgrave MacMillan, 2012.

Phillips, J.: Hermeneutics in psychoanalysis. *Psychoanalysis & Contemporary Thought* 1991, 14: 382–390.

Pinker, S.: *Enlightenment Now: The Case for Reason, Science, Humanism, and Progress*. New York, Penguin Random House, 2018.

Ricoeur, P.: *Hermeneutics and the Human Sciences*. New York, Cambridge University Press, 1981.

Rieff, P.: *The Triumph of the Therapeutic: Uses of Faith after Freud*. New York, Harper and Row, 1966.

Roth, M.S.: Psychoanalysis and history. *Psychoanalytic Psychology* 2016, 33 (Suppl 1): S19–S33.

Roudinesco, E.: *Jacques Lacan & Co.: A History of Psychoanalysis in France, 1925–1985*. London, Free Association Books, 1990.

Rutter, M.: *Genes and Behavior: Nature-Nurture Interplay Explained*. London, Blackwell, 2007.

Rutter, M.: Resilience as a dynamic concept. *Development and Psychopathology* 2012, 24: 335–344.

Rutter, M., Rutter, M.: *Developing Minds: Challenge and Continuity across the Life Span*. New York, Basic Books, 1993.

Samuel, L.R.: *Shrink: A Cultural History of Psychoanalysis in America*. Omaha, University of Nebraska Press, 2013.

Schultz, W.T.: *Handbook of Psychobiography*. New York, Oxford University Press, 2005.

Selden, R., Widdowson, P., Brooker, P.: *A Reader's Guide to Contemporary Literary Theory*, 5th edition. London, Pearson, 2005.

Shorter, E.: *A History of Psychiatry*. New York, John Wiley, 1997.

Shrira, A., Palgi, Y., Ben-Ezra, M., Shmotkin, D.: Do Holocaust survivors show increased vulnerability or resilience to post-Holocaust cumulative adversity? *Journal of Trauma and Stress* 2010, 23: 367–375.

Sokal, A., Bricmont J. *Intellectual Impostures*. London, Profile Books, 1998.

Stannard, D.E.: *Shrinking History: On Freud and the Failure of Psychohistory*. New York, Oxford University Press, 1982.

Twenge, J, Campbell, WK (2009): The Narcissism Epidemic: Living in the Age of Entitlement, New York, Free Press.

Twenge, J.M.: *IGen: Why Today's Super-Connected Kids Are Growing Up Less Rebellious, More Tolerant, Less Happy – and Completely Unprepared for Adulthood – and What That Means for the Rest of Us*. New York, Atria Books, 2017.

Webster, R.: *The Cult of Lacan: Freud, Lacan and the Mirror Stage*. richard.webster.net, accessed November 28, 2017.

Wiltshire, J.: Biography, pathography, and the recovery of meaning. Cambridge Quarterly 2000, 29: 409–422.

Zaretsky, E.: *Secrets of the Soul: A Social and Cultural History of Psychoanalysis*. New York, Knopf, 2004.

Zaretsky, E.: *Political Freud*. New York, Columbia University Press, 2016.

Chapter 9

Belief, doubt, and science

Psychoanalysis, even in its current versions, remains resistant to any serious revision of its theories and its practice. Its worldview threatens to make it more of a system of fixed beliefs, as opposed to a set of ideas that can evolve with the appearance of new data. In some ways, psychoanalysis has come to resemble religious beliefs, cults, or secular ideologies – rather than science.

The philosopher Karl Popper (1968, p. 83) cogently made this point in describing how all-explaining theories can be attractive:

> I found that those of my friends who were admirers of Marx, Freud, and Adler, were impressed by a number of points common to these theories, and especially by their apparent explanatory power. These theories appear to be able to explain practically everything that happened within the fields to which they referred. The study of any of them seemed to have the effect of an intellectual conversion or revelation, open your eyes to a new truth hidden from those not yet initiated. Once your eyes were thus opened you saw confirmed instances everywhere: the world was full of verifications of the theory. Whatever happened always confirmed it. Thus its truth appeared manifest; and unbelievers were clearly people who did not want to see the manifest truth; who refuse to see it, either because it was against their class interest, or because of their repressions which were still "un-analyzed" and crying aloud for treatment.

The culture of psychoanalysis makes it slow to adapt. Candidates in analytic institutes read the complete works of Freud, but are not expected to follow the research literature in psychological science. This system of indoctrination makes practitioners impervious to a wide range of research findings. Instead of promoting integration with science, advocates have referred to its clinical method as "our science", and argued that empirical procedures are not appropriate to evaluate psychoanalysis (Harrison, 1970; Green, 2005). To understand why psychoanalysis found itself in this cul-de-sac, preferring orthodoxy and received wisdoms over evidence, it may be helpful to examine research about belief systems and the roots of rationality.

Why belief is emotional

In the 18th century, the Scottish philosopher David Hume (1739) argued that "passions" (rather than reason) are the most powerful force behind belief. Modern psychological research confirms Hume's view of the supremacy of the emotions. People tend to believe what they want to believe, over-riding contrary opinions and failing to respect facts. As the author and editor of *Skeptic* magazine, Michael Shermer (2011, p. 5) put it:

> We form our beliefs for a variety of subjective, personal, emotional, and psychological reasons in the context of environments created by family, friends, colleagues, culture, and society at large: after forming our beliefs we defend, justify and rationalize them with a host of intellectual reasons, cogent arguments, and rational explanations. Beliefs come first, explanations for beliefs follow.

Our minds are designed to make sense of a complex, often confusing world, by infusing chaos with purpose and meaning. We look for meaningful patterns, and organize perceptions of reality accordingly. Based on a large body of research, two psychiatrists, Michael McGuire and Alfonso Troisi (1998), have suggested that the human search for causality is an evolutionary adaptation for survival, built into the structure and function of the brain.

Psychoanalysis has been particularly adept, rightly or wrongly, at what might be called "connecting the dots". Its theories attribute causality to constructs ranging from drives to early childhood experiences. But these theories try to explain everything about the psyche. Real science raises more questions than answers. Even the most consistently predictive models in the hard sciences must be considered to be provisional rather than final.

Most people in the modern world celebrate the scientific method. Yet throughout human history, people have believed more in *stories* than in facts. The preference for good narratives over solid data has not changed. A story backed by effective rhetoric can overwhelm objections and carry the day. This is part of the reason why the Bible or the works of Karl Marx have been considered to be sacred texts. And classical psychoanalysis is a powerful narrative. It seems to explain almost everything about human nature.

Consider the concept of *psychic determinism* (Freud, 1901/1989), which argues that there was no such thing as a random thought or a random action. This theory is appealing because it offers an explanation for almost any mystery about human psychology. But anyone can speculate, all too freely, about what might be in the unconscious mind. If you become good at this game, you will find little you cannot account for. But even if you create a compelling narrative, you could still be entirely wrong.

Truly scientific ideas are always provisional, presented with a good dose of uncertainty. Investigators always consider that other factors, some of which have not necessarily been measured in research, can be involved. Most research papers end with a statement that since conclusions cannot be firm, further studies are warranted. This preference for doubt over certainty allows for later correction, and is one of the great strengths of the scientific method. It is entirely unlike a system in which the ideas of a founder are taken as gospel truth.

Scholars who have not been trained in scientific methods can go even further astray. More than two decades ago, John Mack (1994), a psychoanalyst and professor of psychiatry at Harvard (awarded a Pulitzer Prize for a biography of Laurence of Arabia), openly defended the claim that space aliens were abducting people on earth to conduct experiments. This bizarre idea was one example of the faddish false beliefs that were used to account for puzzling psychological phenomena in the 1990s (McHugh, 2005). I have heard that Mack had a troubled son who claimed to have had a meeting with an alien, so this false belief could have been an attempt at family reconciliation. Nonetheless, Mack's credulity was extraordinary.

Changing minds

When I was a medical student, I came across an obituary of a scientist who had claimed to have found a bacterium she believed to be the cause of multiple sclerosis. Unfortunately, no one else could find this organism.

What, I wondered, would it be like to spend one's life espousing an incorrect theory based on inaccurate observations? But even among scientists, once one believes something strongly, it is rare for them to change one's mind. Most go to their graves sure that posterity will prove them right.

Not everyone likes to change their mind. As the famous physicist Max Planck (www.brainyquote.com/quotes/authors/m/max_planck.htm) once put it: "A scientific truth does not triumph by convincing its opponents and making them see the light, but rather because its opponents eventually die and a new generation grows up that is familiar with it". In the long run, bad theories are discarded when younger researchers adopt better ones. We can see this kind of generational evolution in psychoanalysis, in which younger theorists are more open to new ideas than their predecessors.

I have been involved in scientific controversies myself. One experience in my research career demonstrates some of the problems. I worked with a psychologist in Vancouver, Kerry Jang, who had carried out large-scale behavioral genetic studies on twins. Kerry and I collaborated on a paper using a scale measuring the capacity to dissociate (Jang et al., 1998). The twin method allowed us to measure its heritability by comparing concordances between monozygotic and dizygotic twins.

That problematic term "dissociation": describes a range of psychological phenomena ranging from feelings of unreality to problems with memory. The reader may think this is an obscure subject, but our research was conducted at the height of a time when hysteria about child abuse gripped parts of North America. As described in Chapter 7, it was claimed that a large number of psychiatric patients were victims of child abuse, but had either "repressed" memories of such experiences, or "dissociated" (splitting their minds) to prevent themselves from remembering them (McHugh, 2005).

These ideas were a return to some of the earliest theories of psychoanalysis (though Freud later backed away from them). The proposal was that "dissociative identity disorder" (i.e., multiple personality disorder) is a common condition that psychiatrists were missing because they failed to use methods to remove repression (such as hypnosis). Dissociation was considered a defense against traumatic experiences, sometimes creating alternative personalities (van der Kolk, 2015).

Our group showed that like all other psychological phenomena, the capacity for dissociation is a trait subject to individual variation related to a genetic influence that accounted for about half the variance (Jang et al.,

1998). Thus even if child abuse played a role in promoting this phenomenon, the pathways to pathology could only be understood as an interaction between a heritable predisposition and life experiences. Today it is widely understood that there no human trait related to personality or psychopathology that lacks a significant heritable component (Plomin et al., 2013). But in getting the message out, we ran into obstacles.

Unfortunately, when I presented the preliminary findings of our research to a meeting of the American Psychiatric Association, I had the wrong results. The graduate student who had been assigned to analyze our data had pressed a wrong key on the computer. As a result, the initial findings failed to show that dissociation was heritable. The assigned discussant for our paper was the Stanford University psychiatrist David Spiegel, a strong advocate of diagnosing patients with dissociative identity disorder. Spiegel was delighted at our apparent failure to demonstrate heritability for dissociation. Moreover, a reporter from *Science News* (a popular magazine put out by the American Association for the Advancement of Science) was in the audience and wrote about our work. This was the only time in my career I was ever mentioned in that magazine – and it was for a mistake. When we re-analyzed the data, it became clear that dissociation, as measured by a standard scale, had the same degree of genetic influence as personality dimensions.

To add to the complications, another psychologist, Niels Waller, a professor in Minnesota, along with Colin Ross, a prominent advocate of dissociative disorders, published a paper (Waller and Ross, 1997) claiming to show that the most pathological aspects of dissociation are *not* heritable (and must therefore be attributed, as they would have it, to the effects of childhood trauma).

When we finally published our corrected results, they showed that dissociation is indeed heritable. Since almost every trait in psychology has a heritable component, we almost had to be right and Waller had to be wrong. But when I shared my concerns with Kerry Jang about how we could convince colleagues, he responded by saying that science was full of contradictory findings that eventually get sorted out. He reassured me that time would tell. And even though Waller and Ross published in a higher impact journal, and were therefore quoted more than we were, few today would support their conclusions.

What actually happened was that almost no one else examined the issue after 1998. One has to ask why. The answer lies in the zeitgeist of research.

Scientists study hot issues that attract grant support and ignore issues that lie out of the mainstream. Over the next 20 years, interest in dissociation collapsed (Paris, 2012). Today, only a minority of therapists still pursue the search for repressed memories of child abuse.

The dissociative disorders (i.e., multiple personality) movement, and the public hysteria that accompanied it, have disappeared. The zeitgeist of psychiatry now favors genetic research, and the idea that dissociation is heritable fits in with the more general view that personality and psychological capacities are rooted in gene-environment interactions. In other words, people who dissociate already have heritable traits that make this phenomenon possible. It is more likely to happen after psychologic trauma. But those who lack this trait will probably never show dissociative phenomena.

A culture of doubt

The worldview of science requires embracing what I like to call a *culture of doubt*. But valuing uncertainty demands preparation and training. It requires mourning for a certainty we all wish for, but that does not exist. Scientists speak of hypotheses that may be disproven, rather than theories, doctrines, or dogmas that are unquestionable. But leaving room for doubt is necessary for progress in science. No matter how tempting it is to find security through sustaining an ideology, doing so contradicts the scientific worldview.

If these principles were applied to psychoanalysis, then publications on the subject would look more like the books of John Bowlby (1969, 1973, 1980), in which empirical evidence is offered to support all theoretical arguments. They would look less like the works of Freud, or other books by psycho4analysts, which spin a story illustrated by a small number of case histories.

Science cannot fully explain the world, but remains the best attempt that has ever been made to do so. It does not claim revealed truth or divine purpose. Its progress is always slow, with more unknowns than knowns. Its conclusions are always tentative and never certain. Science contrasts with ideologies that offer false certainties that deny human ignorance.

Yet scientific theories have often been stubbornly held in spite of evidence that contradicts them. We need to consider some of the obstacles to changing one's mind that affect everyone. Scientists, no matter how well trained, are not immune to these errors.

Why it is hard to change one's mind

Cognitive biases are patterns of thinking that involve errors, distortions, inaccuracies, or irrationality, along with a tendency to interpret reality according to preconceived ideas. Daniel Kahnemann (2011), a prize-winning behavioral economist, developed a model in which the brain uses two systems for making decisions. System 1 is usually applied first, and emotional forces drive these rapid judgments. System 2 is a backup, in which reason can be used for decisions that do not require an immediate response. Strong beliefs generally adhere to System 1. They are based, not on careful reasoning, but on an emotional need for explanation. In the end, any kind of causality feels better than none. Yet intuitions can often be wrong, which is why they need to be reined in by careful reflection. When people are emotionally committed to a belief, it becomes very hard to change minds, possibly because beliefs are linked to emotional circuits in the brain when first formed.

In short, once you make a decision, it is difficult to go back on it or admit you were wrong. Much the same principles tend to apply to any decision in which there is an investment – whether in money, time, moral principles, or emotional commitment. This is called the *sunk cost* problem, in which people justify past decisions by persisting in the same course, rather than revising their choices in the face of new data (Arkes and Blumer, 1985).

Cognitive biases are also referred to as "heuristics" because they function as short-cuts, and are linked to rapid responses. The most important of these is *confirmation bias*, the tendency to only consider information that corresponds to preconceived ideas (Sutherland, 2007). This most pervasive of all biases explains why it is so often impossible to change another person's mind with arguments or facts. If you have already made up your mind, you will only consider evidence that supports an already established point of view. And you will also find a way to dismiss any evidence pointing in a different direction.

Confirmation bias is the key problem with reaching conclusions based on clinical methods alone. If you already have a strong theory in your mind, it will influence the way you hear what patients tell you. It may even influence patients who want to please you to tell their story in line with what they perceive to be your model.

This is why so many therapists with contradictory ideas come to believe that their own theories, and not other people's theories, are strongly confirmed by clinical material. Moreover, if you practice within a community of clinicians who think the same way as you do, you are even more likely to have confirmation biases. And working within a community also supports an *availability bias*, in which people come up with explanations that most easily come to mind (Kahnemann, 2011).

Logical fallacies also influence belief. *Hasty generalization*, i.e., induction based on insufficient evidence, is one of these (Sutherland, 2007). This problem particularly afflicts psychoanalysis, in which practitioners have often been tempted to reach vast conclusions from what their patients say to them. This happens even if clinicians are psychoanalysts who have only treated about 100 people in their lifetime. (I have seen tens of thousands of patients during my own career, but without empirical data, experience doesn't guarantee that my judgments are more likely to be correct.) Freud used this method, but intense interest in the few case histories he published is paradoxical, given that they were mostly therapeutic failures (Crews, 2017).

Moreover, what troubled people have to say about their life experiences, irrespective of their veracity, is rarely representative of the population as a whole, and cannot therefore be the basis of a broad theory of the mind. Research shows a phenomenon called *hindsight bias*: when people are depressed, they remember the past more negatively, but when they recover from depression, they remember more positive events (Blank, 2017). That is why clinicians should be interested in whether their theories of causality can be confirmed by community surveys of attitudes and behaviors conducted by social scientists in large, representative samples.

Finally, clinicians may underestimate the authority they have over their patients. Some research suggests that patients may tend to say what therapists want to hear (Wampold, 2001). That is also why the "tally argument" (Grunbaum, 1984), based on agreement or disagreement from patients, cannot, by itself, be considered a validation of therapists' theories.

In summary, conclusions based on clinical experience alone can be heavily influenced by cognitive biases. And once established, opinions can be resistant to change. Psychoanalysis is a story that is quite dramatic, that catches the imagination, and that suggests a vast web of causal relationships. But no single theory can make sense out of the human condition. To advance both science and practice, we need to embrace a culture of doubt.

False beliefs in clinical psychology

The need for belief is universal, and a universal problem. In my work as a psychiatrist, I often see patients fall victim to illusion in intimate relationships and then suffer from painful disillusionment. Yet these problems are not confined to those who are psychologically troubled. False beliefs are seductive and powerful because they have the capacity to make our lives meaningful.

The loss of belief is also a universal human dilemma. Once we give up on certainty, we can feel grief over the loss of meaning. To outgrow this need, we need to hold a worldview that acknowledges the vast scope of human ignorance. Even now, given how much remains unknown, the world is afflicted by false beliefs of all kinds, associated with religious cults, conspiracy theories, and the denial of facts.

False beliefs in clinical practice can sometimes lead to serious consequences. This danger was exemplified by the epidemic of false memories of child abuse in the 1990s (McHugh, 2005). It was a time when many troubled people, not to speak of some people with normal life problems, became convinced that they must have been sexually abused, but had forgot that such events had ever occurred. Therapists used strong suggestion to convince them that they suffered from repressed memories.

This malignant fad showed how we are more suggestible than we realize. One-size-fits-all explanations, such as trauma and repression, appealed for all the usual reasons, providing simple answers to very complicated questions. Or as HL Mencken (www.brainyquote.com/quotes/authors/h/h_l_mencken.html) once put it, "For every complex problem there is an answer that is clear, simple, and wrong".

In spite of its research base, psychological science has not escaped the problem of false belief. A book by Lilienfeld et al. (2014), now in a second edition, nicely describes some of the pitfalls and pseudoscientific ideas that have afflicted clinical psychology. The problems include false beliefs about the science behind expert testimony, the diagnostic and treatment fad associated with false "recovered memories" and dissociative identity disorder, and the widespread use of psychotherapies that are not evidence-based and/or dangerous. Each of these ideas is associated with pseudoscience, with overly rapid System 1 thinking, and with a failure to apply a necessary level of doubt and empirical testing to ideas that are initially appealing. Each has been associated with a community of believers who have kept scientific inquiry out of the picture.

The psychological mechanisms behind decision-making are relevant to false belief, as shown by studies of medical diagnosis and treatment. Physicians are required to come to rapid conclusions about highly complex problems. This sometimes makes their decision-making process problematic, particularly when they already have cognitive biases that affect what they see (and don't see) in their patients. An American physician, Jerome Groopman (2007), has shown that diagnostic errors in medicine arise from rapid impressionistic thinking and an availability heuristic, as opposed to more careful and reliable procedures.

My own discipline of psychiatry is unusually complex, since much less is known about the causes of mental disorders than about physical illness. Our lack of knowledge reminds me that the less is known, the more tempting it is to adopt false beliefs that provide a sense of certainty. Borrowing from the title of a famous book on pseudoscience by the American mathematician Martin Gardner (1957), I wrote my own book about the "fads and fallacies" that have long afflicted the field (Paris, 2013). Most of these had to do with false diagnoses and unwise therapies.

Those who challenge false beliefs need to make a responsible attempt to apply the same critique to their own ideas. My own beliefs have changed greatly over time. When I trained in psychiatry, there was no guiding paradigm that made theoretical sense out of psychological symptoms. But almost everyone around me, both faculty and students, assumed that classical psychoanalytic theories were a valid way of approaching these problems. To question these conclusions, I would have to have had something to replace them with, which I didn't. It is difficult to question an ideology when surrounded by others who shared it. Thus, even if I never became a true believer, I embraced palpably false beliefs. It took decades before I understood that this was a way of conforming to my social environment. Today much the same can be said about a false belief in psychiatry that every patient with a mental disorder can be managed with some form of psychopharmacology.

An evidence-based perspective is essential for psychology and psychiatry. Yet it contrasts with the way clinical work is practiced. Practitioners want to be sure they know what they are doing, even when they don't. It is worrying that clinicians, who we depend on for our health, can fall victim to false beliefs. But as research shows, finding causality where this is none, particularly when there is an emotional need to find connections, is part of human nature (Shermer, 2011).

Even direct evidence may be ignored if it does not fit one's preconceptions. One famous example in psychology was an experiment in which subjects watching a video of people playing basketball failed to see a woman in a gorilla suit enter their visual field (Chabris and Simons, 2007). In another well-known example, Elizabeth Loftus (1979) showed that eye-witness testimony is highly unreliable, concluding that it should not be considered a gold standard by courts. Loftus has been successful in changing opinion on this issue, reinforced by recent DNA evidence showing that quite a few innocent people are wrongly convicted of crimes based on the testimony of eye-witnesses.

In another famous experiment, on obedience, the American psychologist Stanley Milgram (1974) had his assistants convince normal people to give what appeared to be lethal electrical shocks to people (actually confederates) who supposedly were taking a test. (One of the keys to this degree of obedience was that the subjects had already agreed to give lower levels of shock.)

The study of belief has a large literature, but almost all research studies confirm that opinions are rarely determined by facts and reason alone. By and large, we retain the same religion and the same political views as our parents, our friends, and our social community. Those who dissent will feel the weight of rejection and exclusion. We do not even notice these influences, powerful as they are. We simply assume that what other people in our community think must be true.

The social psychologist Roy Baumeister has proposed that belief fills an essential human need for connection. If shared with others, any belief, even a false belief, can provide a sense of community (Baumeister and Leary, 1995). To believe is to belong, and to give up belief involves separation from a valued community. That is probably why religious beliefs, even those that fall well out of the mainstream, are statistically associated with better mental health.

Leaving the fold of a believing community also means separating oneself from the most important people in one's life. And some religions, such as Jehovah's Witnesses or Scientology, even prevent apostates from having any further contact with their own families. The penalties were less severe for leaving the psychoanalytic movement, but former disciples who split with Sigmund Freud had to pay a stiff price for their resulting isolation. In his autobiography, Carl Gustav Jung (1963) described a brief period of psychosis after his break with Freud. Leaving the movement involved a loss of meaning; giving up strongly held beliefs can irreparably tear the fabric of a human life.

Even in academia, it is possible to live in a bubble of shared beliefs. But unlike a department in a university, a community of believers lives in a closed system. Psychoanalysis created its own societies and institutes outside academia. Its adherents feel they had gained access to a hidden truth, and had insights that the average person lacked. They saw behavior as driven by hidden but powerful forces that could only be understood by those initiated into their mysteries. The movement had sacred texts, popes, and schisms. The process of psychoanalytic training, with its rituals and long periods of sacrifice, resembled preparations for the priesthood. The years patients spend undergoing psychoanalysis, like the pilgrimages of the Middle Ages, reinforced adherence to the cause, creating a body of profoundly committed supporters. But if one makes an emotional commitment to a system that seems to provide definite answers to difficult questions, giving up such a belief means facing a void of doubt. There is only one sure way to protect oneself from false belief. That is the *scientific method.*

The denial of facts that contradict belief is the basis of *cognitive dissonance*, the subject of a large body of psychological research. Thus, when the facts don't fit theory, they may still be molded to support pre-existing beliefs.

Over 60 years ago, in one of the classics of social psychology, Festinger et al. (1956) examined a cult in which the leader had predicted the end of the world on a certain date. But when the world stubbornly failed to end, the members of the cult did not give up their belief. Instead, they found reasons why the anticipated events did not happen when expected, and might still come to pass. In some ways, their fervor was redoubled by disappointment. They came to believe that their prayers had *prevented* the end of the world. (This set of observations is reminiscent of the response of early Christians to the failed expectation of a Second Coming.) While cults fall from the mainstream of cultural belief, the same scenario of illusion and disillusion may be seen whenever people adopt strong beliefs. This is consistent with later evidence that facts rarely change minds, and that people may actually double down on their beliefs (Shermer, 2011).

Since the original report by Festinger's group, nearly two thousand papers have been published on cognitive dissonance. Once people commit themselves to a belief, contrary evidence will be "dissonant" with their assumptions and expectations, and will therefore be rejected. This is one of the mechanisms supporting the retention of false beliefs. One of the predictors of whether a false belief will be retained is whether or not the individual holding it made a significant sacrifice to belong to a group. Leaders will more easily retain commitments when followers do not want to admit they have been wrong.

One can even see the correlates of cognitive dissonance on brain scans. The American psychologist Drew Westen (2007) presented political advertisements to Bush or Kerry supporters at the time of the 2004 American presidential election, and then used functional magnetic resonance imaging to observe which brain areas lit up on. The findings showed that supporters of both parties ignored problematic contradictions, measured either at a mental level, or by fMRI.

In psychoanalysis, evidence that contradicts theory can be accounted for by a complex set of "fudge factors", such as the view that any position can be a defense against its opposite. But cognitive dissonance can arise when psychoanalytic treatment fails to meet its goals. The response is often not to question whether this kind of therapy is appropriate for a patient's condition or to consider alternatives. Instead, one just continues the psychoanalysis – for years, or even for decades.

Psychoanalysis in the 21st century has had to deal with a broader form of cognitive dissonance. One belief was that psychoanalysis is an all-explaining theory of human behavior that does not need to be recreated in the light of psychological research. Another is that psychoanalysis is a unique and effective method of dealing with life problems. To resolve contradictions, some have claimed that analytic theories are too complex to undergo scientific testing. Others state that tests are possible in principle, but too expensive in practice. Still others reject the scientific methods that produce data requiring revision of the model. However, an important minority have accepted that there is a problem, and have made suggestions for revising the model to conform to research evidence (Fonagy, 2004). While not all psychoanalysts have signed on to this project, it is likely that more and more will.

Interminability and sunk cost

Since the time of Freud, a treatment that initially lasted only a few months gradually became "interminable". I have seen many patients undergoing endless therapies over the years. The existence of these "lifers" was documented by a project conducted 50 years ago at the Menninger Clinic in Kansas, in which a large percentage of the patients under study never left therapy (Wallerstein, 1986). Needless to say, this clinic served a very wealthy population. If there is no progress in treatment, one could stop it and consider doing something else. But if there is no defined end-point to the analysis, one can retain the illusion that continuing the treatment indefinitely will eventually yield results. That is why I no longer treat patients in psychotherapy without a defined contract and a time limit.

The interminability of psychoanalysis is a good example of the sunk cost fallacy. People make irrational choices to continue investing their money badly because to stop means admitting that the original decision was wrong. It is hard for people to cut their losses (Kahnemann, 2011). In the case of psychoanalysis, if one has spent five years of one's time (and a good deal of one's fortune) lying on a couch and "free associating", how can one admit the investment may have been lost? (This is not say that one never runs into former patients who feel that analysis did not help.)

The community of psychoanalysts is a binding force for those who remain within the fold. Most of us are greatly influenced by other people's opinions. Surrounded by people committed to the same belief system, individuals find it more difficult to come to independent conclusions. In a famous psychological experiment, the length of a line on a screen was misjudged when everyone else in the room (confederates of the experimenter) presented a different estimate (Asch, 1951). The need for approval by a social group explains why people exposed to contrary opinions tend to dismiss them.

Psychoanalysts, if they had been committed to a scientific culture of doubt, could have practiced their craft with greater humility. They might then have been willing to accept that human psychology is too complex to be understood in a single theoretical model. They needed to be open to emerging ideas from other fields of research. In this scenario, psychoanalysis would, by now, have incorporated the findings of behavior genetics, and accepted that childhood determinism is an over-simplification. It could have also been open to use a wider range of techniques (such as those developed by CBT) to enrich its treatment model. It could have been committed to do whatever makes patients better, not what fits with a heavily invested theoretical position.

It is difficult for clinical practitioners, faced every day with human suffering, to live in a state of doubt. Patients want certainty, and so do their therapists. Of course, psychoanalysis is not the only branch of psychological therapy infected by false certainties. One can see the same process in hundreds of therapies of all persuasions, each of which presents itself as the be-all and end-all of treatment. But as we have seen, the evidence for such beliefs is, at best, thin. The need for certainty may also help explain why psychotherapy integration has had difficulty establishing the same traction as methods that are tagged with a catchy acronym.

Conclusion: a place for psychoanalysis in science

Psychoanalysis, despite serious attempts at revival, still fails to find a secure place within the scientific domain. While some aspects of theory and practice need to be retained, we need to remove accretions accumulated during its history. Only then can we answer the question of whether psychoanalysis will turn out to be a historical footnote, or a courageous but preliminary attempt to understand the human mind.

References

Arkes, H., Blumer, C.: The psychology of sunk cost. *Organizational Behavior and Human Decision Process* 1985, 35: 124–140.

Asch, S.E.: Effects of group pressure on the modification and distortion of judgments. In H. Guetzkow, ed.: *Groups, Leadership and Men*. Pittsburgh, PA, Carnegie Press, 1951, pp. 177–190.

Baumeister, R.F., Leary, M.R.: The need to belong: Desire for interpersonal attachments as a fundamental human motivation. *Psychological Bulletin* 1995, 117: 497–529.

Blank, H.: Recollection, belief and metacognition: A reality check. *Memory* 2017, 25: 869–875.

Bowlby J.: *Attachment and Loss*, 3 volumes. London, Hogarth Press, 1969, 1973, 1980.

Chabris, C., Simon, D.: *The Invisible Gorilla*. New York, Simon and Schuster, 2007.

Crews, F.: *Freud: The Making of an Illusion*. New York, Holt, 2017.

Festinger, L., Riecken, L.W., Schachter, S.: *When Prophecy Fails: A Social and Psychological Study of a Modern Group that Predicted the Destruction of the World*. Minneapolis, MN, University of Minnesota Press, 1956.

Fonagy, P.: Psychoanalysis today. *World Psychiatry* 2004, 2: 73–80.

Freud, S.: *The Psychopathology of Everyday Life*. New York, Norton, 1901/1989.

Gardner, M.: *Fads and Fallacies in the Name of Science*. New York, Dover, 1957.

Green, A.: *Key Ideas for a Contemporary Psychoanalysis: Misrecognition and recognition of the unconscious*. London, Routledge, 2005.
Groopman, J.: *How Doctors Think*. New York, Houghton Mifflin, 2007.
Grunbaum, A.: *The Foundations of Psychoanalysis*. Berkeley, CA, University of California Press, 1984.
Harrison, S.I.: Is psychoanalysis "our science"? Reflections on the scientific status of psychoanalysis. *Journal of the American Psychoanalytic Association* 1970, 18: 125–149.
Hume, D.: *A Treatise of Human Nature*, 1739. www.gutenberg.org, accessed.
Jang, K., Paris, J., Zweig-Frank, H., Livesley, J.: A twin study of dissociative experience. *Journal of Nervous and Mental Diseases* 1998, 186: 345–351.
Jung, C.G.: *Memories, Dreams, Reflections*. New York, Random House, 1963.
Kahnemann, D.: *Thinking Fast and Slow*. New York, Palgrave MacMillan, 2011.
Lilienfeld, S.O., Lynn, S.J., Lohr, J.M.: *Science and Pseudoscience in Clinical Psychology*, 2nd edition. New York, Guilford Press, 2014.
Loftus, E.F.: *Eyewitness Testimony*. Cambridge, MA, Harvard University Press, 1979.
Mack, J.E.: *Abduction: Human Encounters with Aliens*. New York, Simon and Schuster, 1994.
McGuire, M., Troisi, A.: *Darwinian Psychiatry*. New York, Oxford University Press, 1998.
McHugh, P.R.: *The Mind Has Mountains*. Baltimore, Johns Hopkins Press, 2005.
Milgram, S.: *Obedience to Authority*. New York, Harper Collins, 1974.
Paris, J.: The rise and fall of dissociative identity disorder. *Journal of Nervous and Mental Diseases* 2012, 200: 1076–1079.
Paris, J.: *Fads and Fallacies in Psychiatry*. London, UK, Royal College of Psychiatrists, 2013.
Plomin, R., DeFries, J.C., Knopik, V.S., Neiderhiser, J.M.: *Behavioral Genetics*, 6th edition. London, UK, Palgrave MacMillan, 2013.
Popper, K.: *Conjectures and Refutations*. New York, Harper Torch, 1968.
Shermer, M.: *The Believing Brain*. New York, Holt, 2011.
Sutherland, S.: *Irrationality*, 2nd edition. London, Pinter and Martin, 2007.
Van der Kolk, B.: *The Body Keeps the Score*. New York, Penguin, 2015.
Waller, N.G., Ross, C.A.: The prevalence and biometric structure of pathological dissociation in the general population: Taxometric and behavior genetic findings. *Journal of Abnormal Psychology* 1997, 106: 499–504.
Wallerstein, R.: *Forty-Two Lives in Treatment*. New York, Guilford Press, 1986.
Wampold, B.E.: *The Great Psychotherapy Debate: Models, Methods, and Findings*. Mahwah, NJ, Erlbaum Associates, 2001.
Westen, D.: *The Political Brain*. New York, Public Affairs Books, 2007.

Chapter 10

The legacy of psychoanalysis

Psychoanalysis has left an important legacy to psychology. First, it taught a generation of clinicians how to understand the relationship of life experience to psychopathology, and how to listen attentively to what patients say about these experiences. In an era dominated by neuroscience, diagnostic checklists, and overly aggressive pharmacology, patients are not getting the care and understanding they need. We need to find a way in mental health practice to retain a central role for psychotherapy, whose basic principles can be traced back to the work of Freud (Paris, 2017a).

Second, psychodynamic concepts are embedded in all forms of talking therapy, including CBT. Because of the wish to market treatments as unique, the difference between methods has been greatly exaggerated. While there are some specific technical differences (Blagys and Hilsenroth, 2002), similarities, related to common factors in all psychological therapies, are probably more important. In research, head to head comparisons have found few differences in outcome (e.g., Goldstone, 2017).

Third, psychoanalytically oriented psychotherapy now has a very respectable evidence base, but is restricted to treatments that last for months rather than years. This suggests that we can "return to Freud" in a new way – by offering more short-term treatment. As discussed in Chapter 2, the efficacy of long-term therapy for more chronic and complex forms of psychopathology remains uncertain. This book suggests that it should not be the first or the main option when offering initial treatment. In a stepped care model, one might consider reserving longer therapy for patients who do not benefit from a shorter course.

Finally, the concept of psychoanalysis as a unique form of treatment taught in stand-alone institutes has had its day. It is time for the field to re-enter the clinical mainstream. Instead, it should contribute to an integrated and evidence-based model that has one name: "psychotherapy".

My own experience has been that of a psychiatrist who has applied psychodynamic principles within a broader, more eclectic model. Many of my most respected teachers were committed analysts. They were self-confident in their beliefs and strong on rhetoric. But many of their ideas were highly speculative and not necessarily in accord with research. So while surrounded by a climate of belief, I kept my distance. A personal analysis was still a common experience among psychiatrists of my generation, and I found this experience helpful. I therefore remained a supporter, even though I hoped to avoid the narrowness of formal analytic training. One teacher who wanted me to apply to the institute suggested that only by doing so could I "speak with authority". This turn of phrase confirmed my decision not to apply. I was interested in facts, not authority.

After about ten years of practice and teaching, I was dissatisfied with my clinical methods as well as what I was teaching to students. For this reason, I became involved in empirical research. This experience raised even more serious questions about what I had been taught by my own supervisors. Impressed with the evidence for CBT, I added cognitive methods to my clinical tool-box. At the same time, I developed a sub-specialty in personality disorders, for which the most effective methods of treatment involved psychotherapy that combined psychodynamic and cognitive approaches.

Today, when I examine what I do with patients, I regularly make use of psychodynamic concepts. Thus, I am interested in life histories, not just symptoms. I put more emphasis on empathy than on instruction. Most of my practice involves helping patients with borderline personality disorder to manage interpersonal relationships. In this way, the essence of psychodynamic therapy, particularly treatment that uses a relational model, can be distilled, remaining valid and consistent with scientific evidence.

Many aspects of the theoretical paradigm and methods of psychoanalysis can be incorporated into mainstream psychological science. Its principal legacies include the importance of unconscious mental processes, the importance of empathy, and the need to understand and validate life histories. But these principles are currently threatened by mindless practices in medicine, as well as by faddish ideas about psychotherapy.

Psychoanalysis is a humanistic discipline, exploring emotions, thoughts, and behaviors. Unfortunately, humanism in psychiatry (and, to a lesser extent, in clinical psychology) has fallen into decline as reductionistic models have come to dominate practice (Paris, 2017a). Yet one cannot treat most patients with drugs alone, or with manualized versions of CBT. Understanding people and their lives remains essential to all forms of therapy for psychological problems.

Psychoanalysis was one of the first formal forms of psychotherapy. Every method developed since the time of Freud owes something to its ideas. The problem is that while millions can benefit from psychotherapy, most cannot afford it. Classical psychoanalysis is too long and overly ambitious in its goals. While governments and insurance companies fund expensive therapies for cancer and cardiovascular disease, they use research findings to justify the investment. There is a serious lack of evidence for lengthy treatment, a procedure that requires patients to come several times a week for years, and that can only be offered to a small elite.

We need to apply the kernel of truth within psychoanalysis to the care of patients from all social classes and backgrounds. We also need to root these interventions in a broader model of psychopathology. Above all, we need to require that all forms of psychological treatment be evidence-based.

In this light, the rise and fall of classical psychoanalysis can be seen a necessary but preliminary phase in the development of an integrated and evidence-based psychotherapy. Freud could be seen in the same light as Aristotle, whose theories may no longer be considered valid, but who pioneered the systematic observation of nature.

To put it another way, if you practice psychotherapy, you can reject all of Freud's ideas, but as long as you provide a "talking cure", you are, at least to some extent, under his influence. In spite of its faults, psychoanalysis brought humanism into mental health treatment. This is an accomplishment that should not be lost.

We also need to retain certain aspects of psychoanalytic theory. Freud's image of the mind as an iceberg, largely submerged, has been supported by cognitive neuroscience. However, this does not mean, as some analysts would have it, that Freud was right about everything, or as his critics would have it, that he was wrong about everything. One crucial point is that Freud's vision of the unconscious as seething with forbidden desires, or repressed thoughts and emotions, bears little resemblance to what we have learned from research.

Mental disorders are an amalgam of inborn temperamental vulnerability and negative life experiences, both in the past and in the present. This is why many people with childhood adversities can do perfectly well in adult life. Moreover, psychotherapy is most effective when it helps people to deal with current problems. Instead of endlessly reviewing the past, patients need to accept that it cannot be changed, and to develop a future by "getting a life". This is what Linehan (1993) has called *radical acceptance*, i.e., accepting that one's past is unchangeable, but that one can change both the present and the future.

Some of the most thoughtful psychoanalysts are ready to address these questions. This is why I have quoted Peter Fonagy in so many chapters of this book. Similar issues have also been addressed by his colleague, the Belgian psychoanalyst Patrick Luyten (2015). The questions that Luyten sees as important for future research are the theoretical language of psychoanalysis, psychoanalytic technique and training, psychoanalytic developmental theories, object relational and attachment approaches within psychoanalysis, and the nature of general explanatory models in psychoanalysis. In each of these areas, he finds traditional constructs to be wanting, and criticizes the reluctance of the discipline to conduct systematic research that would build a new, more evidence-based framework. As Luyten writes (p. 5):

> Psychoanalysis, as any other scientific discipline, should not shy away from asking these hard questions. It should do so with frank openness and a playful attitude. If not, orthodoxy and rigidity, already widespread in some quarters within psychoanalysis, will lead to a degenerative program of research that will herald the downfall of psychoanalysis as an intellectual and clinical movement.

Gabbard (2010, p. 22), considering the mechanisms of change in treatment, reached a similar conclusion:

> How does psychoanalytic psychotherapy work? Let me state at the outset that the answer is clear – we don't know. Therapeutic action has been much discussed in the psychoanalytic literature, but many of the discussions are inextricably bound to particular psychoanalytic theories. Times have changed; we no longer practice in an era in which interpretation is regarded as the exclusive therapeutic arrow in the analyst's quiver. . . . I have argued that we need to identify what strategies help patients change, rather than worrying about adherence to a particular analytic ideal.

These issues continue to plague contemporary psychoanalysis. Without empirical research, none of the revisions of psychoanalysis will be able to solve these theoretical problems (Grunbaum, 2006). A generation ago, Eagle (1994, p. 404): commented:

> The different variants of so-called contemporary psychoanalytic theory . . . are on no firmer epistemological ground than the central formulations and claims of Freudian theory. Thus, there is no evidence that contemporary psychoanalytic theories have remedied the epistemological and methodological difficulties that are associated with Freudian theory.

Eagle (2014) later noted that for all the discussion about the validity of self-psychology, Kohut and his followers failed to conduct a single research study to determine whether these ideas provided a better explanation of psychological development than classical analysis. In contrast, Eagle (2014) acknowledges the extent to which attachment theory has enriched psychoanalysis. My view is that this model, which has a large capacity for empirical research, could be the best hope for the future of the field. However, attachment theory needs to be integrated with research on temperament to account for individual differences in patterns that cannot be fully explained by childhood experiences.

Again, one of the most important questions facing psychoanalysis, is whether it will continue routinely offering open-ended therapy to all patients, or follow in the footsteps of Freud in his early days, and develop a briefer and better focused treatment. To be fair, the problem of interminability is by no means unique to psychoanalysis. I have observed how CBT therapists, when they do not meet their initial goals, may also go on seeing patients for years. They would be better advised to regularly review the treatment.

At a conference in the 1970s, I was impressed by a behavioral psychologist who began therapy by having both parties sign an explicit contract defining the goals of treatment, associated with a review after a few months to see how well the therapy had addressed them. But when I tried to carry out this exercise for my own patients, I quickly discovered that in most cases I had unrealistic expectations. I now work almost exclusively with patients who suffer from BPD (Paris, 2017b). To say that they have no lack of problems would be an understatement. But I am satisfied if they can give up some of their most destructive symptoms (such self-harm and suicidality). I am also satisfied if they can either get a job or go to school to prepare for one. I do not delude myself with impossibilities, such as a "complete" analysis. The philosophy of my clinical team is that life can be difficult but that one can manage with the right tools. We are not aiming for therapeutic utopia, but are satisfied if our patients increase their level of functioning.

My relationship to psychoanalysis

Like many medical students in my generation, one of the main reasons I chose psychiatry was that I found psychotherapy to be fascinating. At that time, the only real competitor of psychoanalysis was classical behavior therapy, an unimpressive model that tried to explain everything about patients in terms of reinforcement schedules. I trained for two years at a hospital where psychoanalysts were the leaders. While I often disagreed with them, I was impressed with their ability to explain just about everything about patients. Thus I became, with some ambivalence, an advocate for the cause.

Although I was always interested in briefer forms of therapy, I spent many hours in my earlier career seeing patients in treatments that lasted two or three years. My teachers had told me that if you hang in there for long enough, you can solve almost any clinical problem. Since I was working under the generous Canadian health insurance system, money was never an issue. But I gradually realized that this belief was an illusion.

I found that brief focused therapies with limited goals provided more consistent results. I discovered for myself that any treatment lasting longer than six months hits a point of diminishing returns. Eventually I became a convert to a very different cause: *evidence-based practice*. I was no longer willing to carry out procedures that were based on authority rather than on evidence. Unlike some analysts, I did not need to recover from what some have called a "Grunbaum syndrome", i.e., doubt about the truth of the theory and the method (Mitchell and Aron, 2013). It is a mistake to reject the research literature when it fails to support a psychodynamic perspective.

My disillusionment with the form of psychoanalysis I had been taught was painful. I could still treat troubled people, but lacked a consistent model for conducting therapy. But I eventually realized that I could incorporate its best ideas into an eclectic and integrative model of treatment. What helped me was a long-held commitment to applying my medical training by seeing the sickest patients. I gave up using long-term therapy as the primary way of conducing treatment, and in collaboration with some talented colleagues, founded clinics designed to treat patients with personality disorders more rapidly and less expensively (Paris, 2017b).

Yet psychoanalysis left me with a valuable professional legacy. I do not, like too many of my medical colleagues, see all patients as having broken brains that require a pharmacological fix. I learned to understand people with unique stories and with meaningful narratives, and my point of view has not changed. Even when the treatment is not formal psychotherapy, I believe that this perspective makes me a better clinician. There is no substitute for empathy, which is not simply an ability to understand problematic emotions, but puts these feelings into the context of a life history.

The future of psychoanalysis

What will happen to psychoanalysis? In its original form, it is destined to continue to decline. Freud's theory is no longer taken seriously in academic psychology, and its adoption by post-modern humanists does little to help its reputation. Yet some of its most essential ideas can be integrated into a broader model of theory and practice.

The most important of these ideas is that psychotherapy is one of the most effective ways of treating a wide variety of mental disorders. The problem behind the expense and relative unavailability of talking therapy is the continued stigma associated with psychological problems of all kinds (Corrigan, 2004). But it also reflects the reputation of psychoanalysis as an interminable and ineffective procedure.

I expect that the practice of routinely offering patients extended courses of therapy of any kind will also decline. While some cases will always require more time, therapy need not be so open-ended that it becomes endless. In practice, most therapists can manage the majority of cases briefly. But this is not the case in office practices where patients are unusually well insured or can afford to pay full fees.

The problem of treatment without a time limit is not specific to analytic therapy. But there is hardly any research on open-ended treatment of any persuasion. And since studies of this kind are expensive, long-term psychotherapy has never been evidence-based, and may never be. Its use should probably be as more of a backup than a default option.

But these changes can only happen slowly. As Chapter 9 documented, once strong beliefs are held, they can only be given up painfully and gradually. But the older generation eventually disappears from the scene and is replaced by a new generation with different ideas. In a witticism attributed to the physicist Max Planck, science moves forward one funeral at a time.

Not every analyst accepts the idea that most concepts in science and psychology have a shelf life. In a book on the future of psychoanalysis, the erudite American analyst Richard Chessick (2007) imagines (with tongue only partly in cheek) a meeting of an analytic society in 3000. I greatly doubt the movement will last that long. Also, Chessick attributes the decline of psychoanalysis to what he calls a cultural counter-transference. In other words, if you disagree with me, it is your problem. And like many of his colleagues, Chessick doubts whether scientific methods are the most valid way to judge the value of the treatment.

A different assessment comes from the cultural historian Laurence Samuel (2013). Samuel notes that American psychoanalysis benefited from its move away from medicine and into psychology, and that it now has more practitioners than ever (mostly non-physicians). He also observes that psychoanalysis has had a recent vogue in countries (such as France) where it has only recently become popular. But while the ideas behind psychoanalysis remain fascinating to many people, it is rarely practiced in its original form. The media, not recognizing this change, described Pope Francis' therapy in Argentina as psychoanalysis, when it was actually brief psychodynamic therapy.

Jonathan Shedler (2010) has rightly pointed out that while other psychotherapies (such as CBT) are not called psychoanalysis, almost all include crucial elements of psychodynamic theory. To a great extent, Freud can take credit for having initiated the entire enterprise of psychotherapy, including CBT.

Peter Fonagy, in an interview (Jurist, 2010), presented a similar point of view. He sees the future of psychoanalysis as part of an integrated psychotherapy, making full use of CBT and other alternatives, and responding to the demand for briefer treatment.

As of now, it psychoanalysis has evolved, but in the hands of some practitioners, has changed little over time. That is not likely to remain the case. Economic pressures, and the rights of patients to access therapy, require shorter treatment. Meanwhile the movement for evidence-based practice has had a vast influence on practitioners and their patients.

My own analyst, Hans Aufreiter, thought that traditional psychoanalysis need no longer be offered as a treatment for mental illness. The psychoanalyst who was the former head of my psychiatry department, Maurice Dongier, used to tell his patients at the outset that analysis is not a therapy, but a procedure that can provide insight into the mind.

What seems most likely today is that psychodynamic concepts will be integrated into a therapy with a broader theoretical and empirical base. The June 2018 issue of *Psychiatric Clinics of North America* highlights these developments in what it calls "psychodynamic psychiatry: clinical, practical, patient centered, and evidence-based" (Franklin, 2018). And these changes can also be seen in an emerging consensus about how to treat complex mental disorders. John Gunderson, a psychoanalyst who has been a pioneer in empirical research on borderline personality disorder, has come to recommend a once weekly practical approach that uses both psychodynamic and cognitive interventions (Gunderson et al., 2018).

It would be a mistake to reject psychoanalysis because of its all too obvious flaws. It has a core of human understanding that clinicians need, and that I use every day in practice. But, as suggested by Prochaska and Norcross (2014, p. 46), "the future we foresee for psychoanalysis can be summed up by the terms *interpersonal* and *integrative*". It if follows that path, analysis can move out from under the dead hand of orthodoxy. The future must be characterized by an evolution towards being both *evidence-based* and *accessible*.

References

Blagys, M.D., Hilsenroth, M.J.: Distinctive activities of cognitive-behavioral therapy: A review of the comparative psychotherapy process literature. *Clinical Psychology Review* 2002, 22: 671–706.

Chessick, R.: *The Future of Psychoanalysis*. Albany, State University of New York Press, 2007.

Corrigan, P.: How stigma interferes with mental health care. *American Psychologist* 2004, 59: 614–625.

Eagle, M.: The dynamics of theory change in psychoanalysis. In J. Earman, A.I. Janis, G. Massey, N. Rescher, eds.: *Philosophical Problems of the Internal and External Worlds: Essays on the Philosophy of Adolf Grunbaum*. Pittsburgh, PA, University of Pittsburgh Press, 1994, pp. 373–402.

Eagle, M.: *Attachment and Psychoanalysis: Theory, Research, and Clinical Implications*. New York, Guilford Press, 2014.

Franklin, T.: Psychodynamic psychiatry: Clinical, practical, patient centered, and evidence-based. *Psychiatric Clinics of North America* 2018, 41: xv–xvi.

Gabbard, G.O.: *Long-Term Psychodynamic Psychotherapy: A Basic Text*. Washington, DC, American Psychiatric Publishing, 2010.

Goldstone, D.: Cognitive-behavioural therapy versus psychodynamic psychotherapy for the treatment of depression: A critical review of evidence and current issues. *South African Journal of Psychology* 2017, 47: 84–96.

Grunbaum, S.: Is Sigmund Freud's psychoanalytic edifice relevant to the 21st century? *Psychoanalytic Psychology* 2006, 23: 257–284.

Gunderson, J.G., Masland, S., Choi-Kain, L.: Good psychiatric management: A review. *Current Opinion in Psychology* 2018, 21: 127–131.

Jurist, E.L.: Elliot Jurist interviews Peter Fonagy. Psychoanalytic Psychology 2010, 27: 2–7.

Linehan, M.: *Cognitive Behavioral Therapy for Borderline Personality Disorder*. New York, Guilford Press, 1993.

Luyten, P.: Unholy questions about five central tenets of psychoanalysis that need to be empirically verified. *Psychoanalytic Inquiry* 2015, 35: 5–23.

Mitchell, S., Aron, L., eds.: *Relational Psychoanalysis*. New York, Routledge, 2013.

Paris, J.: *Psychotherapy in an Age of Neuroscience*. New York, Oxford University Press, 2017a.

Paris, J.: *Stepped Care for Borderline Personality Disorder*. New York, Elsevier, 2017b.

Prochaska, J.O., Norcross, J.C.: *Systems of Psychotherapy*, 9th edition. New York, Oxford University Press, 2014.

Samuel, L.R.: *Shrink: A Cultural History of Psychoanalysis in America*. Omaha, University of Nebraska Press, 2013.

Shedler, J.: The efficacy of psychodynamic psychotherapy. *American Psychologist* 2010, 65: 98–109.

Index

For Product Safety Concerns and Information please contact our EU representative GPSR@taylorandfrancis.com Taylor & Francis Verlag GmbH, Kaufingerstraße 24, 80331 München, Germany